SEEING
WHAT IS
THERE

SEEING WHAT IS THERE

My Search for Sanity
in the Psychedelic Era

ERICA REX

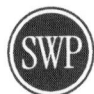

SHE WRITES PRESS

Published in 2026 by
She Writes Press, an imprint of The Stable Book Group

(SWP)

32 Court Street, Suite 2109
Brooklyn, NY 11201
https://shewritespress.com
Library of Congress Control Number: 2025915462
Print ISBN: 979-8-89636-036-0
eISBN: 979-8-89636-037-7

Interior Designer: Tabitha Lahr

Printed in the United States of America

Names and identifying characteristics have been changed to protect the privacy of certain individuals.

For my sister

Andrea Naomi Leiderman
August 8, 1959–September 11, 2005

CONTENTS

Chapter 1

THE DOORS OF PERCEPTION

The day I arrived at Johns Hopkins Bayview Medical Center in May 2012, Baltimore Harbor was not visible from the Bayview campus. A winding road surrounded the grounds and its acres of parking lot. The front lawn sloped southward toward the Patapsco River and Baltimore Harbor, the single green reminder of the farms that once flourished here. To the west, I could discern only the sooty skyline of downtown. I was told that only on the most clarion of cloudless days, mostly in the dead of winter, you might actually catch a glimpse of a moored rig or two. All the same, I wasn't here for the view. I'd come to Baltimore to take part in medical research as a study subject at the Johns Hopkins University School of Medicine's Behavioral Pharmacology Research Unit. In the next few days, I would be taking a dose of psilocybin—the psychoactive ingredient in "magic mushrooms." There would be days-long physical and psychological screenings. The session itself wherein I would receive the psilocybin dose would last an entire day. The process would repeat a month later, in June, when I'd return.

In several experiments held at Bayview as well as other major research universities throughout the United States, cancer patients like myself were being given psilocybin to test the hypothesis that psychoactive drugs provided significant relief to those who suffered from cancer-related depression. Over the course of a few months, with the aid of two guided medication sessions, patients had shown great improvement and had consistently regained a sense of existential meaning in the face of deadly disease.

In the years between my departure from New York in 2009 and the day I arrived at Bayview in 2012, I'd become someone I did not know. My life had receded from me like a tide vacating a storm-wrecked beach. I could not imagine life more than ten minutes into the future. Perspectives right and left narrowed into their vanishing points. I'd experienced this phenomenon before.

During my teenage years, when life at my parents' house descended into real hell, my world became limned within the outline of a keyhole. I had no peripheral vision. I knew something was truly wrong then. What I was doing tomorrow, next month, next year had become abstractions. Plan? What was a plan?

Before cancer, I had been career obsessed. My own career had become derailed in the late 1990s because of a previous major illness. I was married then, living in the Sierra Nevada foothills in California in a small logging town. Endometriosis was debilitating in ways cancer was not. The magnitude of physical suffering it wrought—excruciating abdominal pain, nights spent racing down the mountain to the nearest emergency room sixty miles away, internal bleeding, shock, multiple hospitalizations, a dozen surgeries, a bowel resection, ensuing complications, and then, finally, a total hysterectomy—all that was a world apart. Gone were any illusions I'd had about becoming a mother.

During the time I was ill, my husband had—unbeknownst to me—recommended his cocaine habit. His habit had been a problem in our relationship from the beginning. When I'd found out about it a few months after we'd started seeing each other, I told him to leave. After a while, he convinced me he'd stopped using and was in counseling. I started seeing him again on the condition he was not using. I naively believed he'd quit entirely before we married. It emerged, though, ten years later, he'd resumed. He blamed my illness and the endless hospitalizations. Each time I'd end up in the emergency room, he said, he thought I'd die. Cocaine was his drug of choice to combat anxiety and his own formidable depression, which at times was so severe he refused to engage in any real conversation for days.

After several years of go-rounds wherein I'd leave for a few months to give him a chance to stop, then return, knowing he used a lot more when I wasn't there, he declared the discussion of drugs off the table in any reconciliation negotiations. Even though my endometriosis was more or less cured, overnight menopause had dragged along with it countless life-shellacking hormonal issues. Any faith I'd harbored about the emotional resiliency of my husband's and my dozen-year union evaporated.

I had to leave. Like, really leave. And I was terrified of starting over alone.

Endometriosis did give me one gift, however: an unqualified point of comparison disease to disease. Physically speaking, endometriosis made breast cancer seem like a walk in the park. Breast cancer was virtually painless.

John and I divorced in 2005, and I moved from my home in central California to New York in an attempt to find purchase on the narrow ledge of my journalism career where I'd left off some years before. I lived hand to mouth in some of the sketchier sublet and apartment-sharing situations New York is renowned for. There was the reefer-stoked aging hippie divorcée in Tribeca who turned off my electricity when I would not join her in a project to defraud the city for 9/11 relief funds; there was the dog-faced sixty-something retired schoolteacher who invited friends in for sadomasochistic three-ways during the weekends in the apartment.

I took every editing test in the city—most publishers' default point of entrée, regardless of résumé, qualifications, or experience. I was in my late forties by then. The journalism and publishing world was in an insane state of implosion. No one would hire me.

I struggled from freelance assignment to freelance assignment, from fact-checker to book researcher to travel-guide writer to short-term engagements at major magazines and news organizations to the occasional article. I walked dogs. I worked in a bookstore.

I had health insurance coverage thanks to the California-mandated three years through my ex-husband's COBRA plan.[1] My benefits would expire in 2008, leaving me, unless I could find a job with a health plan, out of luck.

A former friend in California who worked at the local telephone company in North Fork, the mountain town where I'd lived during my marriage, got a certain amount of derisory mileage out of contrasting what my life had become to that of the motivational speaker Elizabeth Murray, whose life story was depicted in the 2003 TV film *Homeless to Harvard*.

"She was 'homeless to Harvard,'" quipped Cheryl. "You're 'from Harvard to homeless.'"

In 2008, barely scraping by, I realized a journalism degree might help. A return to graduate school might provide me a leg up and a few new skills. At least it would give me a peer group, a frame of reference, and some contacts if I was lucky. I applied to Columbia Journalism School, where, once ensconced in a postgraduate science journalism fellowship, I could, for the first time in a long time, start making future plans. It was transformational. The world opened.

Then came the lump. On April Fool's Day 2009, I was diagnosed with breast cancer.

I had gotten to know an Englishman online slightly in late 2008. Despite his exaggerated enthusiasm for the relationship, which existed by dint of Skype and email, my own feelings were wildly ambivalent. All I'd had in mind was something light. No commitments. My career came first. The words *pen pal*, *occasional*, and *transitional* came to mind.

My Columbia University student health insurance expired at the end of August 2009. From the time I separated from John, I'd believed, given the right circumstances, I'd soon be back on the career train with a job, reliable income, and, of course, health insurance. Yet here I was, a middle-aged breast cancer patient without job, family, or government-mandated health care, clinging to the wreckage of the US economy, trying not to drown in the undertow. Watching the Obama administration shovel bailouts at Wall Street was awe-inspiring in the way observation of life itself can be awe-inspiring if you're so engaged, while sipping a vodka martini from your rooftop garden, listening to the Doppler hiss of a world-ending meteor on its final approach. Obama's plan to provide people like me with medical insurance was years away. And even then, I seriously doubted it had any chance of lasting a change of administration.

By the time cancer came calling in early 2009, it was clear the employment world as I'd known it no longer existed. Senior people at major news organizations were invited to retire early or to take career-scuppering buyouts. I could no longer expect the offer of a job. Even with the aid of a Columbia degree and more publications in prestigious newspapers, looking forward to surgery, radiation therapy, and possible chemotherapy, there was no way anyone would hire me. I could make it through surgery and radiation on my Columbia insurance. Copays were going to be another matter.

A bankruptcy lawyer provided me a free initial consultation. It took him ten minutes to tell me I had to be sleeping on a friend's sofa with less than $1,500 in the bank in order to qualify for New York State Medicaid. After that, I was out of luck.

The Englishman proposed an out. By then, we'd met a few times, even spent Christmas together. He suggested we get engaged, and I could apply to move to the United Kingdom via the consular process, which could begin immediately. Under his nominal care, I could move and become a permanent resident, eventually a citizen if I chose. That way, the process would take around three years rather than five, which would be the elapsed time if I were, say, an asylum seeker. In so doing, I would receive ongoing medical treatment through the National Health Service (NHS).

At the time, my feelings veered between numbness, fear, and hysteria. Despite all of my attempts to do what Americans love to tell each other to do every time they encounter adversity—"Pull yourself up by the bootstraps"—I'd run out of ideas. The very notion is ludicrous: People who have no boots also have no bootstraps because they are barefoot. Those who receive veteran's benefits have bootstraps. Those whose entire families have fed at the public trough throughout their lives, like those whose property was bequeathed upon them by the Homestead Act or whose corporations were bailed out by taxpayer dollars, have hefty bootstraps courtesy of you and me. And yet despite the fact I'd always paid my bills, always paid my taxes, voted in every election, was a good friend to my friends, had no criminal record, didn't abuse drugs, exercised and ate healthily, there *were no social supports* to help me in 2009.

My corrosive family of origin had conditioned me to a set of beliefs I had not yet shaken. It went like this: "If your life goes tits up, we will not help you. No one will help you. You are on your own." Both my socialization at the hands of my parents and the twisted values of the postindustrial US political and social hierarchy reinforced those feelings. The rich would be fine. How ordinary mortals were supposed to be resourceful in this surreal rendering of twenty-first-century America I had no idea. Norman Rockwell had disappeared into the realm of make-believe. The United States of America had arrived at full on Hieronymus Bosch.

It took another few years for real rage at the nation that had allowed me to arrive at this place to season. As a Dutch therapist at a breast cancer support organization in London, whom I saw twice a few years later, said the first time I met her without missing a beat, "The American state takes the role of the abusive parent."

Desperation is never the right frame of mind when making important decisions, but it was either take what was available, even if it wasn't exactly my first choice, or throw myself on the mercy of public assistance in the city of New York.

I accepted the Englishman's offer. During that sweltering summer of radiation therapy in Washington Heights, when I could barely stagger home from the radiation suite at Presbyterian Hospital to my studio apartment on Haven Avenue, I managed to sell most of my belongings, pack up what I could not leave behind, and organize transporting my dog, Amalie, into the one country in the world that maintains it has eliminated rabies. I do not believe this, but I wasn't arguing. I arranged for Amalie to have the rabies antibody titer test.

Blood samples are sent away to the single vet lab in the United States that performs it—Kansas State University, in Manhattan, Kansas. Since almost no one ever needs it, the lab waits until they have enough samples to justify the cost of the test. The lead time can be months.

I organized all of her papers for UK customs and the Department for Environment, Food and Rural Affairs. On September 1, 2009, I got on the plane to Heathrow.

I knew the moment I arrived at the Englishman's house in the Midlands near Stoke-on-Trent I had made a dreadful mistake. But by then, the only way out was to keep walking.

It took three years of UK Border Agency interviews, sheaves of receipts and bills proving continuous residence, travel to agency offices in cities like Sheffield, foreign travel restrictions, background checks, the requisite "Life in the UK Test" administered in the attic of the public library in Wolverhampton, US passport pages added and removed, and exorbitant fees for each and every immigration hurdle the Home Office devised. The £8,000 I paid the UK Border Agency over the course of those years was financed with the help of my former husband and my English partner's boss, who was, I can only surmise, performing a humanitarian act.

The good news was my cancer had not returned. That was supposed to be where the story ended. It certainly appeared to be the end of the story for the medical establishment. Their story was the cancer. Their story had nothing to do with me.

As far as my doctors were concerned, everything was going just fine. Three years after I'd left the United States to obtain ongoing medical care in the United Kingdom, the broad perception that my treatment had been a success remained exempt from perforation. I, however, the embodied soul who was not synonymous with "the cancer," could not figure out why I thought survival had been a good idea in the first place.

Both in the United Kingdom and the United States where I had my surgery and radiation therapy, medicine excels at finding cures for disease and saving lives. All that excellence has created a kind of void, wherein treatment of the disease has outflanked the emotional and existential needs of patients. My demoralization is common among cancer patients. We obsess about survival and what the future holds for us.

I told no one about my feelings. To make matters worse, the English have a habit of telling one how one should feel about one's life, given one's circumstances. The word *grateful* kept popping up.

"You should be grateful that you were able to come here and get free care on the NHS," the lady friend of my partner's boss told me one day. That must have been early 2010. I don't believe he'd told her about his £3,000 donation toward my Border Agency experience.

"It was hardly free," I said. "I paid the UK Border Agency over £8,000."

"Well, still," she said. "It's not like your care cost you anything." She added, "That's why the NHS is in such a terrible state. There are too many foreigners coming here for free care."

"I underwent surgery and radiotherapy in the US. I chose not to have chemo even though the NHS oncologist pushed for it. I didn't feel the cost was warranted. The only treatment I get here is Arimidex."[2]

She did not reply.

The Englishman, who also felt I should be fine, took to flouncing out of the house, shouting about my having brought "negativity" into his life, where he just wanted to go for walks, and he'd bought two folding bicycles for us—and I didn't even give a damn! He left, sometimes for weeks. He emptied the joint checking account. Because I was a recent migrant to British shores still undergoing the settlement process with its conjoined wobbly legal status, I was not entitled to have my own bank account. I would not be able to have my own account until I'd achieved the redoubtable status of "indefinite leave to remain." By then, I would have been in the country two full years and each step in the settlement process would have had to go seamlessly. It was not difficult to run afoul of the UK Border Agency at any time, for almost any reason, I learned, including not having sorted copies of telephone bills in correct chronological order when being called to the interview. I watched a despondent Indian couple being sent away with their sheaf of papers because of an evidence gap of a single month. One single receipt. They'd have to go through that particular stage again, including paying the requisite fee of £1,200 a second time.

I had no idea what the Englishman was doing with the £400 per month I paid him in rent. For a while, a bailiff—the UK equivalent of a sheriff's marshal—sat in a car on the road outside the house, waiting for him to return. The Englishman hadn't paid his council taxes for a year. He owed money to everyone—banks, the local council, payday lenders, his coworkers. He borrowed money on an almost-daily basis from his colleagues at work. He consistently ran out of petrol en route. He did not answer his mobile phone.

I began an online search for effective ways to commit suicide. I had saved a small stash of pain medication from my cancer treatment.

A 37.5 centiliter bottle of vodka could also be useful, as was ammonia and denatured alcohol.

On a Saturday morning in 2010, I thought I might be ready. I sat at my desk. Then, I felt someone staring. I turned and saw Amalie, sitting behind me, regarding me fixedly.

What would happen to her if I died?

I'd seen a public service poster for an organization called The Samaritans at Stafford Station one day while waiting for a train. They advertised help for the hopeless. A trained counselor willing to talk anytime, day or night.

I found their number on the internet. I rang. My expectations were not high. I'd never done anything like this before, and furthermore, I was burdened with the prejudice that in order to call a despair phone line, a person should at least be a heroin addict and have an arrest record. I wasn't sure my personal agonies would qualify me to take their time.

Somebody named Jo picked up. We spoke for almost two hours. It soon emerged that she herself was a breast cancer survivor.

That and subsequent return calls to me by Samaritan staff allowed me at least to start talking. I was able to see that my feelings about who I was and what I'd become weren't being reflected back at me. I wasn't someone who had created my absurd train wreck of a life out of something like whim or poor life-management skills. I wasn't to be denounced for having had a life-threatening disease or for having dealt with the consequences by figuring out a way to access medical care, which my own country would not provide. Having been desperate, in Jo's eyes, had not made me a bad person. She saw me as inventive and capable.

My present life situation provoked a relentless anxiety, despite the fact my physical health was much improved. Objective reality about health care and social welfare in the United Kingdom failed to dislodge my emotional state. Rational thought rarely does. Despite its faults, Britain has a social safety net, to which I was entitled. Europeans, including the British, could not, would not, and will not understand how I felt. The resolute fact of social structures to aid people when they need it form the weft of individual belief about survival and human bonds. They are woven into the fabric of society. Europeans understand people develop life-threatening illnesses. They are part of life. The idea neither family nor society will look after one of its members—this does presuppose membership—in her hour of need is so preposterous to Europeans that they simply cannot get their minds around it. Private enterprise is proscribed from profiting by denying care to those who are suffering.

A young man from the Samaritans who rang me back that afternoon suggested I make a list.

"It seems silly, it seems trivial. But it's one way to start tackling things that right now might seem out of control. I even do it myself," he added.

I made several lists that day and subsequent days. The first item: Find a place to live in London. The second: Get my life back.

I moved at the end of 2010 after returning from a reporting trip to California, first to the apartment of a fellow Columbia alumna, then to a share in East London in Tower Hamlets.

Then, in 2012, my three-year mammogram rolled around. Even though I was functioning by all objective criteria, and I was working a lot more, which helped, as far as my outlook on life was concerned, little had changed.

I arrived at Barts and the London Hospital Breast Centre in central London for my appointment. I registered and sat down to wait. The ceiling must have been four meters high and covered in tin. A television yapped in the corner, its shrieking repartee banging off the walls and ceiling unmodulated. The ancient linoleum floor was pocked and streaked. Soot coated the floor next to the baseboards. Pink bunting festooned the walls. There were pink-ribbon pins on offer at the desk. It was horrible. I tried to find a corner to sit in away from the blare of the telly. There wasn't one. A staff member encouraged me to sit down and relax. I said I'd relax if they switched off the telly.

"Not possible," she said. "The other patients like it."

"Ask them if they really mind," I replied. "Then you can turn it off."

She turned on her heel and went back to her perch at the reception desk.

I managed to get through the physical exam and then was sent back to wait in the waiting room for my scan. The television's squawk was so oppressive, I felt as though there were a pink hippopotamus seated squarely on my chest. I couldn't tolerate it. I got up, collected my coat, and headed for the exit.

"Where are you going?" said the receptionist. "Your scan?"

"I'll reschedule," I said over my shoulder. "I'll ring and reschedule." I headed for the stairs.

"Wait, wait a minute," she said, standing also and coming around the other side of the desk.

I hurried down the staircase. A staff member followed me. I pushed open the exterior door of the building and headed to the tube.

Later that day, the receptionist rang. The Breast Centre's pursuit continued that day and the next. With each imprecation to reschedule, I declined more earnestly. *You can have my breast*, I thought to myself. *I'll leave it off for you in a bag.*

Around that time, I'd begun work on an article about some new research coming out of Imperial College, London, one of the preeminent scientific and medical research institutions in the United Kingdom. As a postdoctoral fellow, Dr. Robin Carhart-Harris used functional magnetic imaging (fMRI) to study how psilocybin worked in the brain. Healthy volunteers were given an injection of psilocybin. Then they underwent an MRI brain scan.

Dr. Carhart-Harris focused on two key structural hubs, the posterior cingulate cortex (PCC), a brain region associated with consciousness, and the medial prefrontal cortex (mPFC), a region associated with executive functioning, which includes mental processes such as making plans, decision-making, and moderating social behavior.

The mPFC, located in the front part of the brain, and the PCC, tucked in the middle, participate in the brain's default-mode network, a set of regions whose activity has been closely linked to our sense of self. Research has shown that constrained, ruminative thinking, which is one symptom of depression—it was for me—is associated with hyperactivity and connectivity in the default-mode network.

The PCC and the mPFC tend to activate in concert, like the first violin and the oboe playing in a symphony orchestra. When a research subject is given psilocybin, these functions in the brain become far less synchronized. Although the PCC and mPFC still play together on psilocybin, it is as though the conductor has left the room. The music changes character. If the brain in its normal state is Beethoven's Violin Concerto, on psilocybin it becomes improvisational jazz. The mind no longer dwells on questions limned by the ego, such as "How will I survive if I'm laid off?" or "Is my husband having an affair with another woman?"

Although psilocybin was used as a therapeutic aid in the 1960s, the neurobiological rationale for its use was never scientifically investigated until Dr. Carhart-Harris began his research.

Among many unexpected findings, Dr. Carhart-Harris found blood flow to the PCC decreased by 20 percent when psilocybin was present, contradicting a long-standing assumption that psilocybin works by stimulating these areas of the brain. The PCC and other regions in the default-mode network with which it is associated are critical connector hubs for information transfer and organization. Putting a damper on the default-mode network is like sending the early-twentieth-century telephone switchboard operator working the rural party line out to lunch. The guardian at the cognitive gate stops minding the store for a while. All working phone circuits become available, and everybody can listen to everybody else's gossip, an experience that can be engaging and distracting and can also take a bored local out of her domestic rut.

In terms of the brain, this translates into a less inhibited flow of information between regions. Reduced control on the part of the default-mode network disrupts some of the symptoms experienced by people suffering from depression, among them the narrowing of thought processes and the tendency to fixate on a particular problem.

For cancer patients like me, the inability to remove their focus from the anxiety about the cancer and what would happen in the future was paralyzing. Giving the default-mode network a day off would allow my emotional cage to open a bit and let my mind roam freely.

On the cellular level, psychoactive substances work by altering the way the neurotransmitter 5-hydroxytryptamine (5-HT) or serotonin is transported across brain-cell synapses, the junctions between neurons where neurochemical information passes from one cell to another. Serotonin is one of the major neurotransmitters responsible for modulating cognition, mood, and motor functions as well as the release of other neurotransmitters, such as glutamate, gamma-aminobutyric acid (GABA), acetylcholine, and dopamine. Serotonin molecules bind to specific serotonin cell receptors on the postsynaptic or receiving cell—5-HT_{2A} receptors—causing a change to the cell's electrical state. An electrochemical message passes to the cell, instructing it to excite or inhibit a nerve impulse. When this activation is repeated a sufficient number of times in neurons in different areas of the brain, it alters a person's emotional state, as well as her personality, her attitude, and her ability to make decisions.

Human and animal studies showed the 5-HT_{2A} receptor to be the key player in the neurological effects of hallucinogens. Psilocybin molecules attach to 5-HT_{2A} cell receptors in much the same way as serotonin and antidepressant molecules do, preventing the serotonin molecule from attaching to the cell surface. Structurally, however, the psilocybin molecule has some key differences from the ordinary garden-variety serotonin molecule. In addition to its 5-hydroxytryptamine structure, the psilocybin molecule has two molecular groups that the serotonin molecule does not: a phosphoryl group plus two methyl groups. The difference between the two molecules is like the difference between an ordinary baguette and a Paris-Brest pastry with its sweetened cream, praline, and hints of chocolate. They don't look, feel, or taste the same. Eating both of them involves chewing, swallowing, and digesting. Both provide energy in the form of calories. But in all other ways, they provide a different experience entirely. Psilocybin—like the Paris-Brest—has additional ingredients. These add up to a substantial biochemical difference downstream. Once the psilocybin molecule binds to the 5-HT$_{2A}$ receptor, an uncharacteristic neurophysiological event comes to pass: the psychedelic trip.

Psilocybin as well as other psychoactive drugs cause the talon grip of ego to loosen, and with that, the consciousness of a wider perspective emerges. With ego dissolution comes the freedom to experience the internal world without constraint.

Dr. Carhart-Harris viewed this experience as inestimable for people who are terminally ill. In my interview with him, he told me, "We're all gripped by our self-importance and our perceived place in the world, our ego. Terminal illness diminishes the sense of self and of agency." The existential insights subjects undergo when under the influence of psychoactive drugs and their enduring positive effects make an undeniable case for their use in psychotherapy.

As we concluded the conversation, Dr. Carhart-Harris asked me with whom else I was speaking. He asked if I had spoken to Dr. Charles Grob, professor of psychiatry and biobehavioral sciences and director of the Division of Child and Adolescent Psychiatry at the University of California Los Angeles. Between 2004 and 2008, Dr. Grob and his colleagues carried out the first contemporary clinical study using psilocybin to treat depression in end-stage cancer patients at Harbor-UCLA Medical Center.

I hadn't realized until that moment that psychoactive drugs had actually begun a quiet return to the treatment room.

Using standardized psychological measurements of depression and mood, as well as screening for other psychiatric symptoms, such as paranoia and grandiosity, Dr. Grob assessed twelve patients with advanced-stage cancer. Each was given two doses of psilocybin in a hospital setting a month apart. The sessions were guided, with trained psychotherapists present at all times.

All the patients who took part in the study reported sustained mood improvement and anxiety reduction after the sessions. The effects lasted for at least six months.

The important thing, Dr. Grob told me, was that forty years ago, clinicians working with psilocybin and LSD found that in alcohol-abuse treatment, as well as cancer anxiety, a single treatment session with psilocybin could create a "psychospiritual epiphany" helping subjects to become less fearful, more spiritually aware, more engaged with their loved ones, and able to see their lives as having meaning beyond what they were experiencing in their physical bodies. Not only did the drug diminish patients' symptoms immediately, but it improved therapeutic outcomes for months, even years afterward.

Prior to their almost-worldwide banishment in the 1970s, hallucinogens were prescribed to approximately forty thousand people who suffered from a variety of emotional disorders, from severe depression to end-of-life anxiety to alcoholism. The results showed remarkable promise in helping the majority of them, particularly the terminally ill, overcome pain, fear, psychological isolation, and depression.

The therapeutic benefit of psilocybin lies in its capacity to provide a neurochemical bridge between spiritual guidance and talk therapy. The drug's value depends entirely on the patient's feelings and perceptions during the session and the way he or she processes the memories afterward. Patients who undergo a transcendent peak while taking psilocybin describe it as among the most meaningful events in their lives.

"The drug is a skeleton key which unlocks an interior door to places we don't generally have access to," said psychologist William A. Richards of the Behavioral Psychology Research Unit (BPRU) at Johns Hopkins University. Richards is one of the researchers who successfully treated terminally ill patients with hallucinogens from the early 1960s until 1977, when the work was shut down. "It's a therapeutic accelerant."

Unlike psychoactive drugs, anxiolytic medications such as Xanax help patients only while they are taking them. The effect wears off when the body clears the drug from the system. Patients must repeat the regimen, often increasing the dosage to obtain the same effect. In contrast, the healing constituent of psilocybin lies within the world the drug evokes during a session. Rather than merely dulling emotions as anxiolytics do, psychoactive drugs enable subjects to follow distinctive emotional trajectories, creating space for insights whose touches endure long after the drug effect has dissipated.

"The profession itself forgot about the promise of the early findings," said Dr. Grob. "Forty years later here we are."

His words were amplified by Stephen Ross, MD, principal investigator of the New York University (NYU) Psilocybin Cancer Anxiety Study. He carried out a clinical trial on terminally ill cancer patients at NYU, much like the one that had been carried out by Dr. Grob at UCLA.

"The issues around alcohol addiction and terminal illness are the same thing," Dr. Ross told me. "These are people in an acute spiritual deficit state."

A spiritual deficit state, brought on by the combination of extreme pain and an accompanying sense that life has lost all meaning in the face of terminal illness, destroys patients' ability to manage their affairs or to connect in any meaningful way with loved ones.

Modern medical care isn't designed to manage end-of-life or even life-threatening illness issues, from pain relief to family worries to existential anxiety. Even in Britain, where the hospice movement originated more than fifty years ago, the emphasis is placed primarily on family support, pain relief, and physical and occupational therapy. Psychospiritual issues are swept under the carpet. The abundance of "feel better" messages like the pink ribbons and pink bunting festooning the breast cancer clinic does little more than sabotage patients' true feelings and dash any hope they might have that real emotions—like fear and anguish—are permissible. And if, God forbid, one tries to express such feelings in the presence of a doctor or a nurse, they're more likely than not to be squashed, with encouraging words like "Come now, stiff upper lip" in favor, I imagine, of not upsetting the staff.

"Existential terror in the dying is the most taboo conversation in medicine," said Anthony Bossis, PhD, clinical assistant professor of psychiatry at NYU and that study's coprincipal investigator, when I spoke to him over the phone. "You can count on clearing the room of internists the moment you mention death."

Caregivers and doctors fall back on what they're good at doing: biological medicine and technological interventions. Forget the human being, she's way too complicated.

I asked Dr. Grob if he had any surviving subjects who would be willing to speak with me. He didn't, but he suggested I speak with Roland Griffiths, professor of psychiatry and behavioral sciences at Johns Hopkins University School of Medicine, who had been conducting studies with psilocybin for several years. Dr. Griffiths had an ongoing Phase 4 (safety and efficacy) clinical trial with cancer patients who were not necessarily terminally ill but were suffering from anxiety and depression related to their illness.

I called Dr. Griffiths. About ten minutes into the interview, I said, "Dr. Griffiths, if it's all right with you, I'd like to reframe our discussion. I'd like to take part in the clinical trial."

"Well," he said, "we can see if you qualify."

By the time I went to Baltimore in May 2012, I'd only just moved to my own place. I'd found a tiny, terraced house with a garden in Uxbridge at the end of the Metropolitan line in northwest London. I'd endured the UK immigration machine and had become a legal UK resident. All that was left was a citizenship ceremony and a passport. I'd extracted myself from the survival-threatening machinations of the Englishman, a man in the end who made a point of getting even. Six years on, he managed to connive Lloyds Bank into reopening a joint account I'd had to open with him when I first arrived in the UK, asserting it had never been properly closed. He attempted to create an overdraft for which I would be responsible.

The Bayview campus comprised an institutional jumble of mid-rise edifices whose design, construction, and demolition have been ongoing for about 150 years. The BPRU building, where I was going to be spending the better part of the next several days, was located in a newer part of campus, a building separate from the hospital. The research taking place there was in keeping with the institution's tradition of breaking new ground in medicine and public health.

That work falls outside of the psychotherapeutic tradition. The unit's charter has focused on people and how they live and thrive within society and what happens to people and institutions when the social and physical bonds break. In other words, the purpose of the work is one of broad, public, psychological, and emotional health rather than any specific relationship between therapist and patient. The model is entirely different from what takes place at psychoanalytic institutes and in most psychotherapists' offices. The therapeutic dyad does not exist. Here, it is all about the process.

The messy teardown of one old building known as B Building, an enormous gray art deco structure, dominated the landscape while I was there. The half-demolished brick shell, once part of the original Bayview Asylum, stood amid heaps of rubble. Most recently, B Building had housed patients diagnosed with psychiatric disorders who self-medicated with street drugs or alcohol.

Bayview is part of the massive Johns Hopkins University and Johns Hopkins Hospital and Health System. The facility is at once teaching hospital, world-renowned research center, and clinical medical center. The redoubtable institution as it exists now retains only a faint echo of its humble beginnings.

The hospital started life in the mid-1700s in Baltimore proper as the city's almshouse. Almshouses were a common feature of rapidly urbanizing metropolises of both Britain and the United States during the eighteenth and nineteenth centuries. They were the first social service institutions to offer respite and shelter to society's outcasts. They oversaw a range of services for a diverse group of the disenfranchised, including criminals, the elderly, orphans, alcoholics, and the mentally ill. Yet the Baltimore almshouse offered something most others of its era did not: It retained a staff of trained doctors, pioneering public health care in an era when it was almost unheard of. Its medical heritage lent what is now a hospital among hospitals institutional legitimacy back in a world where almshouses were primarily known as dumping grounds for undesirables.

In 1801, the Baltimore almshouse spearheaded a public health vanguard by administering the first smallpox vaccination in the state of Maryland. This was forty-six years before the childbed fever revelation by Dr. Ignaz Semmelweis, the Hungarian physician and scientist, that doctors themselves were spreading the disease from woman to woman by failing to wash their hands after examining infected patients. And it was fifty-three years before the English physician John Snow identified tainted water from an East London pump as the culprit in that city's 1854 cholera outbreak.

By the mid-1860s, the original almshouse was both outmoded and overcrowded. The city purchased farmland on Baltimore's eastern outskirts to allow for the construction of a larger facility offering improved services, which became known as the Baltimore

Bayview Asylum. The asylum admitted its first patients in 1866. In its airy, uncluttered new quarters, the rural asylum overlooking the port provided its residents respite from the crush of the city and a convenient out-of-the-way location to warehouse those whose families or communities had deemed them unfit for society. The asylum was among the first in the country to accept African-American patients. There was a working farm on the grounds that provided the nineteenth-century version of occupational therapy and needed cash. A preponderance of patients at Baltimore Bayview Asylum suffered from mental illness, which conferred upon the institution a long-standing reputation as an insane asylum.

When I arrived at Bayview, I was not quite insane, but I was not quite sane either. When I pushed open the heavy exterior door of BPRU that Wednesday morning, I was exhausted. I had not slept in days because of my recent move. I had not slept on the plane. The vestibule I entered was more of a guard's station than a waiting area, complete with what appeared to be a building-security control panel on the wall beside the reception desk and walkie-talkie on the counter. I gave my name to the guard who asked me to sign in. Then she phoned upstairs. Through the square, reinforced window on the door behind her I could see a stairwell leading up to the second floor. The guard asked me to wait and gestured to a plastic chair in the corridor. The facility was heavily secured, and comings and goings were strictly monitored, both, I learned, because of the necessity of keeping study subjects anonymous—we're not supposed to meet, much less get to know each other—and because Bayview houses an inpatient rehab center for those undergoing drug and alcohol treatment. Sometimes, as happened one day during my visit, patients chose to leave suddenly, making their way into other buildings.

A young woman with straight blonde hair came down the stairs. She introduced herself as Samantha. She was the research-program assistant who would be supervising my visit. I followed her to the second floor.

Samantha showed me to an alcove sofa, offered me some tea, and gave me a sheaf of questionnaires to fill out. She took my blood pressure, a procedure that was to become a ritual for the next few days.

All study subjects were screened for mental, emotional, and physical problems before they were officially admitted into the study. Before I'd left London, I had filled out several questionnaires designed to winnow out those who might have disorders they didn't know about. There were questions like "Do you ever think there are people or other beings who are transmitting secret coded messages to you alone?"

No, that hadn't happened to me. That question and many like it were repeated several times in different ways over the course of the workup. I learned later why: For people who had underlying psychotic disorders or schizophrenia, the use of hallucinogens like psilocybin could be catastrophic.

Patients in the study visited the Baltimore clinic twice, receiving a low dose of psilocybin on one visit and a moderately high dose on the other. The doses were given blind—in other words, neither the subject nor the guides knew which dose was given during which session.

Later, Mary Cosimano, the study coordinator I had spoken to several times over the phone, invited me into her office, where I filled out even more questionnaires, including assessments of optimism and pessimism, pain scales, depression scales, queries about my lifestyle and my habits, as well as one called Assessment of Spirituality and Religious Sentiments. Mary asked questions about my marriage, family of origin, my life in England, my education, and my work. She asked me about my illness, my diagnosis, and my feelings about my prognosis. I told her about running out of the Breast Centre in London. After an hour, I was crying. She, like everybody I spoke with during my time at Hopkins, had a box of Kleenex tissues on her desk. She asked me if I meditated—I had done some mindfulness meditation—so she suggested we meditate together for a few minutes.

Mary turned out to be a master of three-minute meditation breaks. I took several over the next few days.

Following the interview with Mary, a full-tilt psychotherapeutic dissection ensued. All my feelings and experiences—from childhood trauma to attitude to internal conflicts—were subjected to scrutiny. The guides attendant at the psilocybin sessions themselves have to know the lay of the psychic land so they can be supportive if complex or painful feelings arise during the session. They often do.

The medical workup was equally thorough and included every possible blood test: liver function, white blood cell count, and inflammation factors. The physical exams often uncovered maladies subjects themselves weren't aware of. Borderline diabetes, heart arrhythmia, or slightly off-par liver function would get you excluded, as well as traces of alcohol or drugs. There was an echocardiogram and a neurological workup. I was told later on there have been people who have arrived entirely ignorant they had hepatitis C or a heart murmur. They were sent home.

There were also those who remembered in the middle of an interview—even two days after their arrival—that a grandmother had been hospitalized for something later determined to be bipolar disorder. Even those with second- or third-degree relatives with schizoaffective disorders were considered too risky. I have an asymptomatic clotting disorder, which is treated with low-dose aspirin. The internist who examined me wanted a second opinion. She wanted to be sure that psilocybin, which sometimes causes an increase in blood pressure, was not going to be risky for me.

At the end of the day, I had my first meeting with Roland Griffiths.

There was a bit of Ichabod Crane about Roland, who was tall and thin and had a head of pure-white hair. He wore enormous glasses. His gaze pierced. His demeanor together with the hair and his temperate, methodical way of moving made me think of a loris. His office decor consisted entirely of caffeine in various manifestations. There was a picture of hands holding a coffee cup; and some old Coca-Cola posters. Roland spent years studying the long-term effects of caffeine on the brain.

I'd spoken with Roland at length on the phone. He'd emphasized before we'd even agreed I'd come to Baltimore that I could not take part in the psilocybin study if it were going to be just a journalistic exercise. For the purposes of the study, which was both expensive and complex to conduct—the foundation underwriting the research had paid my airfare and was paying the lion's share of the hotel bill—my participation would become invalid if I were merely observing. Furthermore, if I were to maintain a deliberate emotional distance, my likelihood of having a bad trip would increase.

I reiterated that I had not come as a journalist. I'd parked journalism at Heathrow Airport. I'd handed in the scientific article before I left London. It dealt solely with neuroscience discoveries Dr. Carhart-Harris had made during the course of his psilocybin research using magnetic resonance imaging. Though his work and his scientific discoveries were fascinating and far-reaching in their implications, its journalistic import could hardly be considered riveting. I was there as myself, as someone who was upset and anxious and depressed because of everything that had happened since my cancer diagnosis three years before.

Roland's concerns were not just verbal choreography around how a game of table tennis ought to be played in the interest of creating an optimally sporting experience. They had to do with the essentials of "set and setting," key factors in the hallucinogen-assisted therapy equation.

"Set" refers to "mindset"—the subject's mental and emotional attitude toward the hallucinogenic experience. "Setting" is the physical and social environment—the room or the space itself and the people who are present with the subject during the experience.

Part of the "set and setting" reckoning includes the ability to have complete trust in the guides, trained psychotherapists who remain with the subject throughout the entire session. The images and feelings a person experiences can be beautiful and transcendent or terrifying and disgusting—or all of these over the course of the day.

"Radical curiosity," said Roland. "That's how you have to approach this."

His message was clear: If the current of the experience carries you downriver, metaphorically speaking, do not resist, just go with it. Engage with the trip and why you're going. Struggling toward shore will get you nowhere. The subject's "set" had to include a willingness to move toward repellent or frightening thoughts and images, rather than trying to avoid or fight them. When you arrive at a precipice, you have to allow yourself to plummet over. Or submit to capture by the fugitive slave catcher. Or get eaten by a bear.

Roland talked a lot about "ego." Part of our conscious mind comprises an ego, the sense of "I" as separate and distinct from other people or beings or objects in the external world. Ego is the mistress of our individuality. Normally, ego is the element of mind that keeps a person from jumping off the real-world cliff just because it might be an interesting experiment in weightlessness. Ego forms the basis of our instinct for self-preservation.

In the psychedelic therapy setting, if ego tries to keep the experience at bay, its interference will run athwart the entire process. Where ego can't or won't get out of the way because of a lack of trust and transparency, bad trips often result.

Those who carried out therapy with psychoactive drugs during the 1960s and '70s and who are engaged in these projects today have a mantra: "Trust, let go, be open." Some study subjects have a very hard time doing this. Most of us who were raised in the United States over the last two generations have a hard time relinquishing control.

On one occasion at BPRU, a study subject resisted the experience to such a degree that he fled the session room and had to be coaxed back. In another case, the patient became so terrified and so resistant during the induction phase (the period of time when the drug starts to have an effect), he panicked. The guides had to restrain him physically and reassure him until he could once again "trust, let go, and be open."

Toward the end of our meeting, Roland told me he knew my elder sister, D. Over the decades, I'd periodically googled my siblings. I knew D was a neurologist and had worked for at least two federal agencies, the National Institute on Drug Abuse and the Center for Drug Evaluation and Research. I knew before I arrived it was very likely she and Roland had crossed paths professionally. I was not surprised, I told him. I knew it was a risk. He quickly dismissed any notion their acquaintance was a risk. He told me they'd served on a few boards together. They were not friends, he assured me, and they did not see each other socially.

He repeated, "It's not a risk."

I am not sure he understood my response. Perhaps he was concerned I doubted his professional integrity.

Far from it.

I knew Roland himself would never betray confidence or breach privacy. Such conduct would be unbecoming to his profession and unbecoming to the conduct of anyone in the medical or psychotherapeutic community. What he did not yet know was that I had to take his integrity as an article of faith. I had to believe his character did not bear any resemblance to that of my parents, their peers, and members of the medical and psychotherapeutic fields with whom I'd been acquainted over the years.

More than once, I'd heard my parents talk openly about matters told to them in private by their friends, by their own children, as well as by their patients. They discussed freely what others would consider confidences, mentioning subjects by name. My father bragged openly about having seen the poet Anne Sexton in therapy in Boston for a short while when her regular psychiatrist was away. He spoke of her in terms at once misogynistic and licentious, taking credit for a book she was working on while under his care. He bragged about giving tapes he made of their sessions to an English professor at Stanford, who later wrote a book about Sexton.[3]

It was like listening to someone revel in a tale of intimate grand larceny or rape.

In the 1980s, I cut all ties with my family of origin. My decision did not sit well with my parents. They persevered in tracking me down despite my moving repeatedly and changing phone numbers. Eventually, thinking I was not making my point clearly enough, I penned a letter letting them know the relationship was well and truly over. I had already begun therapy with a clinical social worker, Chet Villalba.

Rather than giving rise to the mature self-assessment or introspection one might at least hope to see from trained psychiatrists, the letter just incited them further. They contacted my friends, former employers, and doctors. They even managed to locate me by way of my automobile registration after I'd moved to the mountains.

My parents expected everyone they knew—and even those they didn't—to collude with them. In describing me, I later learned, they laid out a narrative of unalloyed psychosis. D contacted the attorney I'd retained to write cease and desist letters and tried to coerce him to work with "the family" as a go-between. That D could be oblivious to the law and the corresponding code of ethics she so blithely breached could seem far-fetched to those not familiar with my parents' approach to interpersonal maneuvering. In the context of "the family," it made a bit more sense: Both she and my brother glided like sleepwalkers through my parents' burnished confabulations. My brother showed up at my house one day unannounced, I guess to haul me in. I didn't open the door.

A very old friend from childhood told me she'd encountered D at a high school reunion. Tearfully, D maintained she did not understand why I was doing what I was doing. She'd read a personal essay I'd written published on the Web. She wanted to know why I was writing such terrible, horrible lies about "the family."

"The family" to me represented nothing more than a cult, the kind that grows up around narcissists, psychopaths, and cult leaders—toadies who are terrified of what the narcissist will do if he finds out someone thinks he's wrong or flawed. Toadies who stand to reap a material reward.

Trusting Roland and the process was a decision I'd made before I even got on the plane. It was going to be one of the "set and setting" tasks for me. Trust, let go, be open. I knew from what I'd read and from speaking with him that Roland was not interested in creating power relationships. He was not a man of the twentieth century's misogynistic psychoanalytic school. Roland was interested in humanity and spirituality. Roland wanted to talk about ego, of course, but he mostly wanted to talk about God.

"What do you think about God?" he asked me that first day. "Where do we go when we die?"

I had no idea how he expected me to answer.

Roland himself was a serious meditator. He'd taken part in several silent meditation retreats, ten or more days each time, in meditation for ten hours each day.

Over the course of the two-day workup—a tryout to see if I would actually be accepted into the study—I spoke with four psychologists and researchers. Mary interviewed me for hours. One researcher, Dr. Matthew Johnson, who was studying smoking cessation using guided psilocybin sessions, asked me during our interview, "If you had to spend the day being nauseated, could you tolerate it?"

I suspected nausea was going to be the least of my problems.

I had true emotional rapport with Chet, yet my feelings toward most people in the field were—and are—largely negative. My sensibilities did not spring fully formed out of nowhere.

In my experience, there are too many people whose wholesome nature I'd call into question who have entered the professions grouped under the umbrella of "psychology." I'm in no position to speculate about how or why people choose any given profession. But I am, whether I like it or not, cursed with an innate ability to see errant therapists for what and who they are the moment I meet them. They appear before me like dystopic *commedia dell'arte* harlequins. They may as well wear motleys, carry wands, and sport hook-toed slippers decked with bells. They are counter empathic. They caricature empathy. I've been told since by a woman intuitive that there's a name for this dubious gift: claircognizance. I simply know too much about people, just by being in the same room with them.

Thursday morning, one of these lurched into the picture.

I arrived for my scheduled appointment at ten. Mary accompanied me because the social worker I'd be meeting was not a senior Hopkins researcher but rather a trainee doing his internship, which meant he could not meet with subjects or patients unsupervised.

We waited expectantly in an office. The trainee, introduced as Dan, finally arrived late, flustered, perspiring, in a flurry of motion. He sat down and without hesitating or making eye contact started pulling papers out of his folder and flapping them onto the table in front of him.

He leaned back in his chair and crossed his legs.

"Tell me about yourself, Erica. What brings you to Baltimore? What brings you to Hopkins?"

I looked at Mary, who explained that Dan had been briefed about my background but wanted to find out a bit more about me in my own words.

I recounted, as I had done now several times over the past twenty-four hours, what had happened since I was diagnosed with breast cancer and left New York. He interrupted me mid-sentence.

"One of your questionnaires says something about horses. Do you still ride?"

"No, I don't," I replied. "I can't afford to. I haven't since I left California. I sold my horse in 2004."

"Why?" he said.

"Well, I don't exactly have that life anymore, my life has changed a lot, and—"

"But why not, if you enjoyed it?" he interrupted.

I looked at him.

"Because my life changed. I changed countries. I lived in New York, then I left New York, and now I live in London."

"Yes, but you could have ridden in New York, right?"

I glanced at Mary, who had pasted a look of benign disinterest across her face.

"I was broke. I moved to England for medical care because I could not afford care any longer in the United States. I am a breast cancer patient. That runs my life now. Why would I be in Baltimore in the first place if I weren't a cancer patient who wanted to be in the Hopkins study?"

"Right," he said, as if it were the first time he'd heard of it.

I looked down at my hands.

"I don't know how they choose guides, but I hope you're not going to be my guide," I said, "because it won't go well."

Dan's face turned crimson.

"I am trying to find out why you would stop doing something you liked doing, that's all," he said, implying, I can only surmise, I could take more responsibility for improving my own life.

"I don't know what to say," I said after a few moments. "I've said repeatedly I couldn't afford to ride or keep a horse anymore, not in New York, not in England, not anywhere. I've tried to answer your questions and yet you interrupt me and keep repeating the same question over and over. I have no other answers." I paused. "And I really couldn't see going into a situation with someone like you where I'd have to be self-revealing."

"I think Dan is trying to get a sense of how your life was before you had cancer," said Mary.

"I have nothing else to say," I said.

The meeting ended quickly thereafter.

Back in Mary's office, she wanted to talk about my reaction to Dan. The discussion devolved into a paradoxical and circular discussion about my honesty—which was evidently considered a good thing—while my reaction to his antagonistic ineptitude was certainly not.

Still jet-lagged and still having not slept since I arrived forty-plus hours before, I was so tired and burned-out by then, I could not stop crying.

"If this is about pleasing someone who doesn't know what he's doing, then I should go back to London," I said. "That would be fine with me, really," I said.

"No, no," said Mary, handing me Kleenex. She suggested we meditate for a few minutes.

Later that morning, after I'd returned to BPRU from the clinical medical wing where I'd gone for more tests, I met with Roland again.

"I have to tell you, we were concerned about your reactivity to Dan. We're worried about whether you're a suitable subject for the study."

"You want me to leave? Sure, no problem."

"It's not that," said Roland. "It was your extreme reactivity in that situation."

"Some guy who is supposed to be a psychologist fires questions at me in an interview room and interrupts me when I try to reply. He asked me three times why I don't ride anymore. He ignored my responses. I'm supposed to sit back and smile and take it? You've got me coming and going, Roland. I'm perfectly happy to leave right now if this is how it's going to be. Really."

"Okay, this is administrative, and technically not your concern, but I think I should tell you," said Roland. "We confronted Dan about what happened this morning because he had some answering to do for how it went. He said he was flustered. There had been a traffic jam and he was stuck in traffic, which is why he was late. He owns his behavior."

"I see," I said, "and as the somewhat compromised person who came all this way, I have the privilege of paying the price for his traffic jam and abominable clinical skills. That is rich. Makes me feel right at home."

I could not control my tears. Roland handed me the Kleenex box.

"Here's the thing. When you're in the session, you can't fight it. We say, 'Trust, let go, be open.' Ego can't get in the way."

"If I'm being attacked by an 'ego' in the present tense, I defend myself," I said. "If he or anyone like him is going to be the guide, I'm not the person for this job."

"He isn't a guide. He's a trainee social worker," said Roland. "I'm not talking about Dan. I'm talking about being able to trust the situation with your guide. You have to trust the person and the situation. Trust, let go, be open," he said, repeating the mantra again. "We should talk after you spend time with Fred."

"Who is Fred?"

"Your guide. Depending upon how it goes, we'll make a decision. You'll meet with him later this afternoon, and then all day tomorrow and Monday."

"Okay," I said. "But if I feel as badly tomorrow afternoon as I do now, I will leave. I can call the airline this afternoon. I don't need this." I stood to go.

"Let's see how it goes," said Roland. He stood also. Then he came over and gave me a hug.

Besides my questionable capacity to trust, let go, and be open, there remained an unresolved concern about my clotting disorder. Roland had not heard back from the consultant hematologist.

I went to the alcove to wait for Samantha to take my blood pressure. I leafed through books about spirituality and books of pictures. I stared at the beautiful renderings of psychedelic imagery and photographs of the natural world. I thought about times I felt okay in the universe.

That afternoon, Roland introduced me to Fred Reinholdt, who would be my guide. We headed into an empty office.

Fred was tall and loose-jointed. His presence, even the way he moved, was wakeful and open and perceptive. His face conveyed a kind of buoyancy, which I'd now characterize as mirthful. I had the sense of someone inhabiting the world as an integrated soul, fully incarnate, living in his skin without squirming. Fred was also a meditator. From what I learned about him over the next several days, he'd arrived at meditation after years of searching for a spiritual practice that worked for him. His spiritual journey really began, he said, "when I finally decided to take up the cushion."

The spiritual-journey theme recurred several times during those days. As the woman who became my support person and met me at Bayview after the session, Nancy-Bets Hay, herself a counselor at a cancer support organization in suburban Baltimore, put it, "People don't choose spiritual journeys. The journey chooses you. The journey carries you along and you can't dictate how it moves forward."

That afternoon, another emotional evisceration got underway. The singular difference was Fred himself. He already knew a bit about me from speaking with Roland and Mary and Matt. He told me if I wanted to ask questions about the process, or about him, or anything at any point, I was free to do so.

Later on, we moved to the session room—a regular hospital room, to be sure, but decorated with shelves of books, sculptures, and pictures of mushrooms. Lit with incandescent table lamps rather than the overhead fluorescent lights characteristic of most hospital rooms, the space resembled a lounge. There was a sofa in lieu of a bed; there were numerous books of photographs of the natural world. Mushroom imagery dominated the decorative scheme. A swish audio system was set up to play a carefully curated music track during the session, throughout which I would wear headphones and an eye mask. The eye mask was *de rigueur* in these sessions, as a way of helping the subject turn toward the interior world. An automated blood pressure monitor would take a reading several times an hour. Fred pointed to a small, unobtrusive video camera concealed on a high shelf. The sessions were recorded for legal reasons.

We rehearsed what would happen on the day of the session. Fred started up the music track. I lay down on the sofa with the eye mask and headphones on and closed my eyes and meditated for a few minutes.

Friday, we met in the session room again. This time Fred was joined by a woman named Porche, who would be my second guide. There were always two, a man and a woman. Again, we went over aspects of my life, many of which I was visiting for a second and third time since my arrival.

At the end of the afternoon, Fred and I went to speak with Roland. As we waited in the hall outside of his door, I was overcome with apprehension. I was tempted to flee. Fred asked me how I was feeling. I confessed to extreme unease, which had nothing to do with the prospect of taking a psychedelic drug but rather because of what had transpired during the process of getting to this moment right now. I was intimidated by Roland and emotionally undone by the very fact that I had been reduced to a state of vulnerability I had not experienced in years.

"How about this?" Fred said. "How about handing over your anxiety to me for a little while. I'll carry it into the meeting for you and then it will be off your hands. And it won't make any difference at all to me. Anxiety doesn't weigh anything," said Fred.

I looked at him. The idea was ludicrous and inspired. He held out his hands.

"Okay," I said. "Here you go."

I handed it over. Fred took the anxiety in his hands. Then Roland opened the door. We entered and sat down.

Roland asked me how I was doing.

"I was apprehensive and nervous," I said. "But then Fred said he'd carry my apprehension for a while. So I gave it to him. He's carrying it now. I feel okay."

"That's great," said Roland. Then he smiled for the first time since I'd met him.

We chatted a bit more, and then Roland asked me to wait in the alcove.

A bit later, Fred emerged. "Think you'll be ready by Monday afternoon?"

"So I've passed the test?"

"If you want to call it that, yes. How do you feel?" asked Fred.

"I'm fine," I said. "I'm happy I won't have to undergo another day of emotional flaying. I wouldn't last." I asked about the clotting disorder. A second hematologist had been found and consulted. The path led forward now free of obstacles.

There was one thing, though, that stuck in my craw—the matter of the negative scrutiny over my defensive response to the trainee. Fred listened attentively.

I'd had way too much experience with psychiatrists—from my family of origin to therapy to the decades of not being believed by those to whom I told my story. Psychiatrists covered for each other; in so doing, they'd damaged my life and the lives of generations of women.

"Roland, you, and the Hopkins trainee do not know me better than I know myself," I said. "I will not allow a psychiatrist to abuse me narcissistically to protect himself from his own bullshit. Again. Ever."

"If it's okay with you, I'd like to mention this to Roland," said Fred when I was done. "You feel you're being dissed because of your life experiences, which are authentic. I think he should know that."

"If you want to talk with him about it that's fine," I replied. "But if it's going to get me evicted from the study perhaps you should tell him now before the weekend, so I have time to change my ticket."

"Roland has already left for the day. And it won't. The decision has been made. I value your opinion. I can speak for him in saying he also values your opinion."

Monday was much like Friday, spent in the session room with Fred and Porche, talking about my life, and getting used to the mask, the music, the headphones, and the automatic blood pressure cuff huffing away to itself throughout the day. The six-hour music compilation progressed over the course of the session. No track was repeated. The opening tracks consisted mostly of liturgical music, dissolving gradually into classical selections, then world and ethnic music. Then, at the end, "Here Comes the Sun."

Late in the day, I met again with Roland, who had yet more to say about ego and letting go.

"Ego," he said, "wants to prevent us from having this experience. The last thing ego wants to do is dissolve. It will do its best to throw up all kinds of obstacles because in the material world, we need ego for our survival. So, what is the best way to counteract ego when it gets in the way?"

"Trust, let go, be open?" I said.

"I've suggested to subjects if you get to a scary place, something really terrifying, you ask whatever it is that's scaring you, 'What do you want to teach me?' You might even get an answer. And once you ask, you stop being scared. If you approach ego for what it is, the fearful image or experience moves away," said Roland. "Does that make sense?"

In its own weird way, it did.

Then Session Day finally arrived. I was brought into the now-familiar room. There was a vase with a rose in it on the table.

Subjects were encouraged to bring photos and memorabilia to look at and talk about before the psilocybin took effect. Some people had brought rugs, hangings, even sculptures, redecorating the entire room for the day. I'd brought photos of my younger sister, who had died of metastatic colon cancer in 2005, as well as pictures from my former life in the mountains of California, when I was married. I'd brought photos of my horse, my dogs, the landscape, wildlife, all things that meant a lot to me.

The actual administration of the psilocybin capsule was done ritually—as part of the set and setting equation and also to make sure the study's protocol was being followed. Roland came into the session room to give me the capsule and watched to make sure I drank the entire cup of water. Then he left.

I sat on the sofa and shared some of my photos with Fred and Porche. Fred suggested I look at a few pictures in one of the books. Then my head began to feel heavy. I lay down under the sheet and put on headphones and the light-blocking eye shade.

I found myself at a bus stop, getting on a bus. A youngish woman standing near me realized she was on the wrong bus and was shocked and upset by it. She wanted to get off. I was taken aback by her intensity. I thought to myself, *Buses do go both ways.*

Then John came into the picture, not as a distinct physical presence but as an emotional being. I had a sense of how distraught he'd been during my illness and how I had been so absorbed with my own pain I had been unable to be compassionate toward him. I started to cry.

A friend who was something of a connoisseur of the psychedelic experience told me later this often happened to people during the induction phase. Feelings of profound sadness or profound fear arise when the ego starts to dissolve. As far as dissolution was concerned, Ego would prefer not to.

"Those tears are payment to the ferryman who takes you to the other side," he told me. "He'll ferry you across, but he always exacts a price."

A few moments later, I noticed a young boy with a slingshot standing a few yards in front of me. He steadied his arm against a tree trunk, his elbow resting on a branch. He aimed straight at my forehead and pulled back the rubber band. I stared at him, unfazed. I thought, *Gosh, if this is supposed to scare me into not wanting to go ahead, the effort is rather pathetic.*

Beside me there was an explosion. A blinding white light erupted geyser-like out of an aperture in the earth.

Then the notes of a violin solo lit three strands of deep red light, which trickled like water in my right visual field. Deeper tones poured from above in huge blue clouds in the middle distance. Another violin flourish turned the sky yellow and brought with it a comet's tail of body parts flying from the upper left of my visual field to the lower right, disappearing behind me.

Sometime later, I found myself inside a steel industrial space. I became aware of my feelings toward my two living siblings. A woman seated at the end of a long table, wearing a net cap, white clothes, and working busily, turned and handed me a Dixie cup.

"You can put that in here," she said.

So I did. The cup filled itself with my bilious, sibling-directed feelings. "We'll put it over here," she said, and placed it on a table at the back of the room. Then she went matter-of-factly back to work, along with numerous busy women who occupied this space.

Up until then, I had not shared anything at all with my guides. I was completely absorbed by the experience.

Some subjects interact with the guides more than others. Some want to share a bit too much, which can detract from the internal journey and is gently discouraged.

For me, the process was so interior and so compelling, I had not even thought of sitting up and talking about it.

Then Fred asked me if I'd like to share what was going on.

"What a lot of busy women," I said, sitting up and removing the eye mask, as though the irony of their presence was obvious to everyone. As I recounted the scene, I began to laugh out loud, and then Fred began to laugh, and my own laughter appeared to me in a midnight-blue, cloud-dark sky as an effusion of twinkling gemstones, glittering rhythmically with my peals of laughter.

Late that afternoon, I returned to what Roland termed "consensual reality." Mary, Roland, Fred, Matt, Porche, Samantha, and Nancy-Bets gathered with me in the session room for a debriefing. When I told them about my own laughter at the busy women setting off a fountain of jewels issuing forth from the universe, Fred said, "Let that be a lesson to you, young lady."

During the session, the subject of cancer did not arise. Other parts of life appeared and revealed themselves in myriad ways: the present, the past, people known, people loved, and people reviled.

The session defies description in the logic of everyday language. It is impossible to force the literal world onto the experience, even to try to characterize it in terms of a narrative progression or distinct lessons learned.

There was logic to my experience, to be sure, but it was internal and *sui generis*. Unlike some other subjects, I did not have a peak or transcendent experience. I had hoped to see the face of God, and I did not.

Those who have undergone the psychedelic experience and attained what is commonly thought of as a transcendent peak describe it in explicit terms: a sense of oneness with the universe, a complete sense of dissolution of self and being part of something magnificent yet ineffable.

I did not have the distinct sensation of being part of all things and one with the universe, although I had hints of it—the blinding-white geyser, the jewels welling out of the sky symphonically with my laughter. Where I would have expected each of these parts of the experience to effloresce infinitely until the universe revealed itself in its entirety, each image or scenario simply ended or was elided by something else.

I told Fred and later Roland that I was disappointed.

Both pointed out it was an experience that could be neither dictated nor controlled. That, so it seemed, was part of the lesson and part of the journey.

A day later, while I waited at the airport for my flight back to London, I spoke on the phone at length with Dr. Anthony Bossis, the NYU cancer study's coprincipal investigator. He'd given me his mobile telephone number for use if I thought speaking about the experience afterward would help me process it.

I told him about my disappointment at not seeing the face of God.

"This may not be satisfying, but truthfully, these experiences are like peeling an onion. You don't get there until you're ready to. You'll get there, through whatever the modality when it's time."

What I have discovered since about my experience is that it couldn't be placed within the definition of things that count as "cures." It was more akin to the rituals found broadly in indigenous groups, where the psychedelic ritual, in fact, originated. The psychedelic encounter has more to do with shared values and cultural symbolism than it does with biochemistry. What happens in an effective psychedelic experience with the necessary preparatory and integration sessions is not a drug treatment. It is a hero's journey: There's the voyage out; barriers and obstacles encountered; signposts and guideposts recognized; lessons learned from overcoming challenges; the integration of the experiences; and then, finally their meaning and messages incorporated into everyday life.

The Hopkins sessions were only the beginning. For me, they provided a kind of petal-strewn pathway to a different way of gaining self-knowledge.

But, as with all roads, once a person starts heading down them, the rose petals vanish fairly quickly, to be replaced with uneven cobbled surfaces often riven with potholes, unanticipated hairpin turns, black ice, even improvised explosive devices. No matter how outlandishly huge the growing pharmaceutical hype becomes, the dangers are all there, and increasing numbers of people are going to encounter them.

Chapter 2

THE FOREST AND THE PATH

Unlike active-duty combat veterans, my emotional condition did not result from military service. I was not there on 9/11 helping terrified people out of the burning buildings. Nothing about what happened to me was noble or ennobling.

My emotional troubles came about because I was the child of my parents. Was I unwanted because I was born too soon, a mere seventeen months after my elder sister? Did my gender disappoint? Perhaps a male second child had been expected. This was the theory of one psychiatrist—a former trainee of my father who was trying to explain away my parents' behavior—whom I saw for a total of two sessions. I was simply the wrong child.

From a vantage point of forty-plus years hence, I can say now it was not my business to know. What I do know is that I was regularly beaten from the age of three.

It took me a decade of therapy during my late twenties to late thirties to finally remove the locus of blame from inside my own body. What happened to me wasn't because of who I was or something I did. It was something done to me.

I was the child of a psychologist mother, who was a lifelong alcoholic and the director of a school for autistic children in Palo Alto, and a psychiatrist father, whose personal elixir tended toward medical drugs coupled with fine wines. He was a professor at Stanford Medical School from 1963 until his retirement in the 1980s. Both parents claimed to be experts in the field of child development.

For decades, my father was in charge of selecting which medical school graduates would be admitted to train in the psychiatric residency program he oversaw. He chose men like himself: misogynistic, unhappy in their marriages, resentful of their burgeoning responsibilities, who, once done with their residencies, left the wives who had put them through medical school for sexier, younger women. My father, however, did not leave. Instead he had affairs, and later traveled abroad for extended periods without my mother.

My parents spent their lives entirely within and among the greater Stanford-campus academic enclave. My parents' intimates were white, mostly Jewish, overeducated, and arrogant. The Stanford campus and those who lived there sheathed themselves in armor of inculpability.

A sense of immunity persists in these kinds of communities, no matter what anyone does. Take the priesthood, for instance. It's taken fifty years or so for the crows circling the church to come home to roost. My parents and their peers possessed the same uncanny ability to glide above any kind of moral scrutiny.

My parents—especially my father—also enjoyed a generation-specific postwar, God-given benediction, a consecrated hall pass for the mighty and untouchable. My father would live long enough to be told, over and over, that his was "The Greatest Generation." My parents distanced themselves from the people who lived in more diverse communities like East Palo Alto, Milpitas, San Jose—towns that have changed a great deal in the last half century. Violence in those other communities could be pointed at and derided. Blame could be attributed to race, ethnicity, and social class. That stuff happened elsewhere.

My parents' chosen professions provided them with additional protective coloration. The facts my family of origin presented to their colleagues as well as to my teachers and doctors was that I, as their second child, was the family problem. Were it not for me, everything would have been perfect. My presence alone created trouble. In other words, I was the official scapegoat.

I prefer the French term, *le bouc émissaire*, the emissary goat upon whose back the sins of the community—or family—are piled. Said goat, when banished into the wilderness, carries the filthy burden away with it. Gone and forgotten. Pray that *le bouc émissaire* does not one day return bearing the truth.

She's back, and here's the truth: The psychoanalytic tradition's original sin—and I include modern psychology—is built into the DNA of the profession. My parents' actions lay within an institutional pattern of abuse and cover-up that started the day Sigmund Freud, the father of psychoanalysis, renounced his seduction theory in 1897.[1] Since then, the psychoanalytic field has denied childhood trauma and emotionally annihilated the lives of countless women and children. The labels of "hysteria" or "neurosis" or "just plain crazy" create a twinkly scrim over the terrible reality of suffering. The dangers presented by psychiatry are part of the DNA of the field. Michael D. Cornwall, PhD, writing for the website Mad in America, characterizes psychiatric diagnosis as a "status degradation ceremony" in which psychiatry has granted itself the moral authority to vitiate anyone by diagnosing them, labeling, deriding, nullifying anyone who questions their authority. I call this "naming the scapegoat."

"Psychiatry," writes Cornwall, "is a cult whose leaders turn the protestations of harm directly onto their victims."[2]

The field itself, though, has continued to barrel forward decade after decade, gathering layer after layer of self-justification, lie after toxic lie.

During his brief tenure as projects director of the Freud Archives (1980–1981), psychoanalyst Jeffrey Moussaieff Masson unearthed previously unpublished letters Freud had written to colleagues describing reports of traumatic abuse and molestation among his female patients. At first, compassionately, he believed them. Then, pressured by his peers, members of the Society for Psychiatry and Neurology in Vienna, he rejected his own ideas. Drive theory was born. The real incest, which actually occurred, was transmogrified into the Oedipus complex, a deranged fiction about infantile fantasy requiring yearslong psychoanalytic interventions that generally led nowhere. It was an epic gaslighting project designed to protect the perpetrators. Facts about what had actually happened to his patients, and to all psychiatric patients for the next five generations, were officially banished.

Masson's subsequent publication of Freud's previously undiscovered letters—which had been deliberately omitted from previous volumes by Freud's daughter, Anna—outraged the psychoanalytic establishment.

When I spoke with him, Dr. Masson said, "The problem with the profession was you had to tell women they weren't abused. Nobody in the profession cared if it made sense or not." He added, "Not one of those psychoanalysts is ever going to face what they did. They created more than a hundred years of misery for women. The world has changed. The field has not."

As a very young child, I was forced to conclude that my parents beat me because they had no choice. I was bad. I believed that what happened to me at my parents' hands was my fault. They had to punish me because of what I had done to them: The very fact of my existence made them victims.

In my thirties, I attempted to conjure up events from my childhood I could describe as "normal." Normal was my Ouroboros, a symbol of transcendence from ancient Egypt: a serpent curved into a loop as it consumes its own tail.

The Ouroboros represents the eternal cycle of renewal. Round and perfect, like a merry-go-round ring. Only the very lucky ever bagged one.

If you were blessed and clever—and especially if you had a long arm—you could stretch out your forefinger as you capered past on your wooden steed and pluck the ring from the holder set on a pillar at the ride's edge. The ring earned you a triumphant second round, a sort of victory lap for normalcy.

Summer. A beach. Florida. My sister and I are parked at our grandparents' Miami apartment. I'm about three; D is four. My grandfather sits in his folding chair in the shade of a coconut palm, reading a newspaper. There is an overpowering scent of coconut suntan oil. Our bodies are basted with the stuff. Our skin gleams like slabs of ham broiling on a spit.

The sun's rays bore no danger back then.

I watch two older girls clad in pink-and-red two-piece bathing suits play with a red-and-yellow celluloid beach ball. They stand in the water, ankle deep, and play catch. Back and forth. Suddenly a gust of wind lifts the ball skyward. It hovers, then drops into the ocean. D and I watch it bob on the blue swells for a few minutes. The girls jump up and down and shout and flap their hands. The taller girl runs out a few yards into the water, until the tops of the waves splash at her waist. She puts a hand to her brow, turning this way and that, scanning the horizon. Then she turns and looks back at her friend. She lifts her palms up in a gesture of helplessness. She makes her way back to the beach. The other girl kicks at the knee-high breakers lapping at the water's edge.

We watch the waves carry the ball, farther and farther out until it's just a little red spot. It bobs into view every few seconds. Then it is gone. The two girls stand together, watching. They are crestfallen. The ocean has robbed them of their joy. My grandfather looks up from his paper. Then he looks down again. I think, *Maybe someone will get them a new one.*

We stay at my grandparents' beachside apartment most of that summer. My parents had gone to Europe to do something important. My brother must have gone with them as a babe in arms.

When it's time for us to leave and return to our parents, my grandparents take us to the airport. Our care is allocated to Eastern Airlines for the flight back to Boston. Although she flew with us on the way out, my grandmother will not personally oversee our return to Boston. Unfortunately for D, until this moment, she has not realized the plan was for us to fly back unaccompanied. At the gate, a stewardess clad in a little blue suit and a little blue cap meets us. She greets my grandmother, she proffers both hands, all set to lead us onto the plane. D contemplates the smiling lady's outstretched paw for a second or two, an unnatural thing, tipped with perfect hot-pink-polished nails. No one in our world wears fingernail polish. D backs away. She starts screaming. She does not want to go with the lady in the blue suit, her platinum hair so shellacked and shiny it mimics the gleaming sunlight on the silver sides of the airplane, poised on the tarmac already, preparing to depart. Its engines rev and roar, its propellers turn, the air stinks of diesel. The stewardess grabs D's hand—dumbly, I have already let her take mine—and says to my grandmother, "Just leave and they'll be fine."

Fine it isn't. In the end, my grandmother accompanies us back to Boston. When we arrive, our parents are not exactly happy to see us. They are in a rage. Because of our sniveling cowardice, they were forced to pay for my grandmother's second round-trip ticket. They would become destitute because of us. Do we think other kids would have treated their parents this way?

By the time we return from Florida, we have been separated from my parents for several months. I've started calling my grandmother "Mommy." No one has objected to this nomenclature during the summer—or if they have, they haven't done so with much conviction. Not enough to make me stop, in other words. On our return to Boston, everyone calls my mother "Gloria," except for D, who calls her "Mommy." Since I now call my grandmother "Mommy," I figure "Gloria" is the best name for this new person—whom I recognize, mind you. I just do not know how she fits into the picture.

My phraseology around parenthood does not please my mother. On the drive home from taking my grandmother to the airport for her flight back to Miami, my mother stops at a light and hooks her right arm over the seat. D and I sit side by side in the back. No seatbelts back then. She looks me in the eye.

"I am Mommy," she says. "That other lady who just got on the airplane is your grandmother. She is not your mommy." I stare at her, not quite able to understand why "Mommy" has just left, and yet now "Gloria" is "Mommy."

"You're angry at me for leaving. That's why you're calling me Gloria. I know you. You're angry."

A few months later, my little sister is born. Within the year, I am sleepwalking, when I sleep at all.

It is 1990, and I have been in therapy with Chet Villalba for about three years. I do not know whether I trust him. We talk for an hour twice a week.

Chet and I talk about work, which I hate. I claim I have nothing else to talk about. Chet tries to get me to talk about my feelings toward other people and toward family. He encourages me to articulate my inner life using a color palette containing something other than black dismissives and meaningless extremes, such as "I hate" and "What the fuck do I care?"

Talking does nothing for me. Talk is an exercise in cleverness: intellectual, externalized, and abstract. *Words, words, words,* I think to myself on my way home from sessions. Nothing connects with anything.

I tell Chet repeatedly that, whatever my problem may be, talking won't fix it. I have a physical problem, I say. I, myself, am not really sure what I mean. I'm no hypochondriac with invented maladies. In purely medical terms, I am fine, although I suffer from crippling migraines, which have landed me in the hospital numerous times. I experience a periodic ache in my left forearm, which manifests itself whenever I feel endangered by people—at that point in my life, an almost daily occurrence.

About the time I start seeing Chet, a new class of psychotropic medication has landed on the pharmaceutical scene: selective serotonin reuptake inhibitors (SSRIs), known primarily by their most oft-prescribed brand name, Prozac. Broadly advertised and infinitely gossiped about, they are touted as the best thing to happen to medicine since the polio vaccine. They are the miracle cure for depression, anxiety, and despair, a veritable antidote for humanness itself.

Chet does not suggest I take them. He knows better. I view psychotropic drugs with about the same affection as I do the pretty pink flowers in *Invasion of the Body Snatchers*.

Although not informed by any scientific knowledge at the time, my sophomoric notions about neuropsychiatric medication in general, and SSRIs in particular, are not entirely off the mark.

Chet knows I have cut off contact with my family of origin. He sort of knows why. He asks me about how I feel about my family.

"I have no idea what answer you're looking for. I don't know what you want me to say," I reply.

"There is no right answer, really," he says.

I say, "I feel nothing toward any of them."

I have demurred on the details of my childhood because I am afraid if I tell him, he won't believe me. I've been doubted before.

During a conversation I had shortly before I started therapy with Chet, I'd tried to explain to a friend from grad school about why I thought my relationships during my twenties had been so chaotic, so full of struggles and betrayals, and so fraught with insecurity. S was from Oregon. She hailed from the most stable and loving of families imaginable. She was smug and self-satisfied and had perfect straight blonde bangs. I envied her enormously.

Her reply, when told what happened in my parents' house during my childhood and teens, was quick, adamant, and pitilessly simple.

"You must be hallucinating," she said. "Your parents are pillars of the community."

The friendship ended there.

S's words echoed those of a therapist I saw briefly in my twenties. Mrs. Miller's home and office were located, eerily, in the same Boston suburb where my family lived during the years when most of the violence took place, Waban. She was also a psychologist married to a psychiatrist. When I told her about my childhood and teens, she said, without a pause, "You believe your mother didn't love you." Then she orbited her hands around each other, the same gesture my mother made when she was trying to explain to a teacher or mother of a friend what a misbegotten creature I was, and why I had to be picked up early from kindergarten to go see a psychiatrist twice a week.

"You have an 'imago' of your mother," she said. "Your perception of your mother is not who your mother is. Your mother probably loved you very much."

I should have walked out of her office right then and there and never returned.

My failure to acknowledge my feelings to Chet—or admit that I have any feelings at all—is not doing me much good. I have told him about Dr. Nemetz, the psychiatrist I was sent to as a child, because at the time, I believed that Dr. Nemetz was the single adult who brought order into my family's otherwise out-of-control world. Dr. Nemetz's presence in my childhood forced my parents to behave like grown-ups. Mostly. For a few years, until we moved to California, he was the cop. Except I cannot resolve having been abandoned by him, a conflict I have never discussed with Chet. I remain true to a personal and irrational narrative: He was the single, blessedly good adult who saved me from familial hell. Chet refers to him as "The Good Doctor."

Dr. Nemetz, I now realize, was hired as a decoy, a cover for my parents on the off chance their obsession with destroying me was ever observed by outsiders. Dr. Nemetz could vouch for my insanity. He would declare my parents blameless victims of a child monster.

Now in my thirties, however, my wishful and gilded narratives about people are not serving me. I am often wrong about people. I fall into and out of friendships with women I don't trust. I can tell I'm in danger with people by the sensation in my left forearm, but I have no clue how to avoid these situations in the first place. I cannot read the advance cues people invariably provide—or if I read them, I immediately censor myself for judging people. I start a love affair with a married man who is supervising a project I'm affiliated with. The situation causes me enormous pain. It does nothing for my professional credibility. Chet makes it plain he thinks the choice was a stupid one. He promises he will continue to support me regardless of where the escapade takes me. Chet tries to guide me into talking about my feelings by asking me how I feel about our own therapeutic relationship. This sends me into a fury.

"What the hell does it matter what goes on in here, how I feel about anything in here, in your office? This is a fake situation. It has nothing to do with the real world."

Sometimes, after outbursts, I flounce out of his office. He waits patiently for me to come back in. Sometimes I do. Sometimes I don't. One day, on a hunch, he follows me outside. He finds me sitting in my car. He asks me if I think I might like to go back in. He waits. After a while, I agree to go back inside.

Waban, a middle-class Boston bedroom suburb. I am four years old. D has started first grade. I fear sleep. I have terrible nightmares. Sometimes I sleepwalk and waken elsewhere in the house.

In the living room. In my sister's room. I often force myself to stay awake, drawing or making up stories under my blanket. Sometimes, when I am really scared, I walk down the hall to my parents' room as quietly as I can and stand next to their bed. Sometimes, they wake up and take me back to bed.

Sometimes, terrible things happen.

I pad down the hall quietly and enter my parents' room. Tearfully, at their bedside, I try to explain the nightmare to my parents.

My father awakens first.

"Who is it?"

My mother's eyes float open, and she sees me.

She throws back her covers and leaps from their bed. The smell of adults in the nighttime is both pungent and malodorous—familiar yet infused with the sour smell of something unknowable. My father leaps to his feet, too, and strides around the end of the bed, over to her side. He hoists me to his shoulder. Barefooted, he descends the stairs to his in-home office. I gaze upside down at the backs of his bare heels as he hurries into the office. My father always wears Jockeys to bed. My mother, wearing a thin nightgown—I can see her breasts through the diaphanous cloth—follows, then closes the doors, two solid wood doors, built back-to-back, the way all psychiatrists' doors were built back then to attenuate sound. My father deposits me and I tumble with as much resistance as a sack of flour onto the black-and-white wool-covered couch. He switches on the buzzing fluorescent light. To this day, I cringe whenever I see lights like those, relics from the era of the nuclear family: brown oblong metal things emitting a chemical smell along with their unnatural bluish, headache-inducing light.

I am paralyzed with fear. My mother's blows descend on me—randomly, haphazardly, now on my back, now on my bottom, now on the back of my neck, on my forearm, which I have managed to twist around behind me in an attempt to protect the bare small of my back. My pajama top is rutched up around my chest, and my skin is exposed. Her closed fist thuds against it. Then perhaps because he sees her not being effective, not making the difference a real parent should make, my father pushes her aside. He grasps my arm above the elbow, forcing me face downward against the sofa. I can barely breathe. He pounds on my bottom and thighs and the small of my back first with his open hand, then with his fist closed. My father is not one of those men who limits his outward expressions of anger to shaking his fist at the sky and railing like Job about his victimization by the universe, although he does that too. When he hits, when he yells, he means to inflict pain. Because he is stronger, his blows are harder and they hurt more. My mother's blows and chastisements are haphazard. Often when my mother hit me, I felt she didn't know whom she was really mad at. Hands that ought to stand for comfort—mother's hands—that had held and rocked four children by then, are able to extinguish trust in the time it takes to draw a breath.

Then, suddenly, I break. As though outside of myself, I hear myself screaming, "I hate you, I hate you!" at the top of my lungs. My words are muffled by the cushions. I scream them in the midst of otherwise incoherent sobbing. In them, I am lucid. Otherwise, I have ceased occupying anything I could identify as an integrated body. I am borderless, elsewhere. It is the first time I find myself in the dissociative universe, a space at once terrifying and threatening and then later familiar—the space where nothing hurts anymore and no one can touch me.

Everything halts. My father's blows stop. For a moment, I have stopped life—I have interfered with the parental dynamics as I know them.

My mother sits down on a chair.

"Do you really hate me?" she asks.

My father loosens his grip on my arm so I can move. I do not move and I do not answer. My face is pressed into the woven wool strands of the sofa cushions.

"Answer your mother," says my father. He waits, a Second World War first lieutenant, standing in readiness against four-year-old me, the danger, the enemy. I feel him waiting for me to turn, to look at them, to reply.

"Answer your mother," says my father again. Turning the slightest bit, I can see him now. He stands now a foot or so away from the sofa's edge with his arms folded.

"You don't really hate us, do you?" asks my mother.

"Look at your mother."

I don't move.

"Turn over and answer your mother."

I turn, hiccupping. Tears streak my mother's cheeks. She pulls a tissue out of her nightgown sleeve—she always stuffs tissues into sleeves—and dabs her eyes. I try not to look at her.

My parents have a phrase with which they ridicule me whenever I cry. "Crocodile tears," they would say. "You're crying crocodile tears."

Who is crying crocodile tears now?

"Answer your mother."

"I want to go to bed," I say.

"Tell your mother you love her, and you can go to bed."

Silence. A few remaining tears, spasmodic hiccups on my part.

"Did you hear me? Tell your mother you love her or else I'll really give you something to cry about." He unfolds his arms and shifts his weight, and I know there will be another pounding, another onslaught of fists against my skin.

I make my first survival bargain with the devil. I decide the only way to get away from them is to lie.

"I love you," I mumble.

"What was that? Say it so your mother can hear you."

"I love you," I say. I know I am lying. Eventually, they let me out of the office. I decline my mother's offer of being tucked in.

That night, I learn my first lesson about lying to save myself.

The next day, I am kept home from kindergarten. That day, the day after, and the day after that. Mostly, I am confined to the office waiting room, separated from my siblings by the double doors. Sometimes I hear D outside, asking my mother if I will ever get to go to school. I'm let out for meals and to go to the bathroom. Little fingertip-shaped bruises dot my upper arm. My thighs, a jumble of abstract blue marks. I cannot see my bottom.

Looking back, I have thought at times I knew why they kept me home and separated me from my siblings. Perhaps they worried they'd be found out. Perhaps some teacher or other parent would have noticed the bruising, my depressed demeanor, my inability to make eye contact with anybody. Maybe D would accidentally spill the beans. I could fantasize—and I did at times—that a cast member from the idyllic childhoods being lived by other children might do something to help.

One could hope.

One would have been kidding herself.

Years later, in my early thirties, when I finally had the courage to open the door in my head where the memory of that night and others like it lived, the thing that upset me most was not the violence. Nope. It was my complicity with my parents against my four-year-old self. I called my old boyfriend from Brown University, someone I had really loved but been too scared to marry. At the time, I was terrified of anything that resembled family, which, being a decent sort of guy, was exactly what he wanted. Long before I encountered the screeds of psychoanalytic theory, I intuited them: My biggest secret fear was that if I got married and had children I would turn into my mother. I would be an alcoholic. I would abuse children.

R had spent a few vain years during our twenties trying to figure out what was wrong when it came to trying to love me. Eventually he gave up in frustration and married a girl he'd known in high school. At the age of thirty-two, I recounted my long-closeted childhood story over the phone to him on the other side of the country, sobbing inconsolably because I had aided and abetted. In the strange compression and inversion of time that happens when I revisit trauma, I was possessed of the idea that somehow my adult self ought to have had the wherewithal to protect and save the four-year-old. I had shirked my responsibility.

"But sweetie," he said, "you were a baby. You needed your parents to survive. What the hell else were you supposed to do? You can't judge yourself as an adult. You were a baby, for Christ's sake."

That week, my parents start taking me to a progression of psychiatrists—all with soundproofing and double doors. They settle on Dr. S. Joseph Nemetz in Brookline.

On our first meeting, my mother explains to Dr. Nemetz that the real problem with me—and the reason we were in his office—was that, simply put, since I was born, I had been an out-of-control child. I didn't behave the way other children behaved. I didn't sleep well. I kept my parents and siblings awake. Furthermore, I am violent. I hit my brother, who is a few months shy of two years my junior. This makes her furious.

She tells Dr. Nemetz she fears I'll harm him.

"I have to discipline her," she says. "If she's bad, I have to spank her."

Dr. Nemetz asks me whether the family has rules. I tell him that we don't have any rules because my parents do not want to be strict, like some parents are. He asks me if I think this policy is fair. Both my parents are quick to intervene, to qualify, to rationalize. They follow the child-rearing advice of Dr. Spock, they explain. Dr. Spock advocates against rules.

Later, I came to understand my parents' relationship with rules: They believed in rules for everyone else. They did not believe in rules that were inconvenient to them. They themselves existed above the plane of rules.

In that first session, with my parents, Dr. Nemetz imposed a rule: There was to be no hitting in the family. My father, who already knew on some level that family life was entirely out of control, agreed it would be adhered to. My mother must have agreed in principle, perhaps with her fingers crossed underneath her purse.

From then on, I visited Dr. Nemetz twice a week. We played pickup sticks, Chinese checkers, and marbles. Playing games with a grown man was the stupidest activity I could imagine. I'd rather be at home with my sisters.

It is 1961, a late-spring afternoon. I have been seeing Dr. Nemetz for several months, maybe a year. For a few hours a week, life is stable. I know what to expect.

I have awakened early from a nap and have crept down the stairs. My big sister, D, is in first grade and not yet home; my brother is still upstairs napping. Andrea's playpen is set up in the dining room. She spends way too much time there. A substantial yellow swinging door separates the kitchen from the dining room. Andrea sees me and pulls herself to her feet. She has only recently started walking. She starts to say something to me in baby talk. I want her to be quiet. I don't want my mother to know I am awake and downstairs. Andrea fusses, then squawks, her chubby round fingers clutching the bars of the playpen. Her blonde head barely reaches the top of the rail. I go to the teak sideboard, stand on tiptoe, and reach up for a little carving—a wooden statue, maybe five inches high, that my father bought in Germany on some trip—of a bespectacled doctor in a white coat holding up one finger as though admonishing a patient. A little caption in black writing on the carved pedestal reads: *Einer von uns ist verrückt.* (One of us is crazy.)

I go over to the playpen. I propel the little statue along the rail. I tell Andrea the little statue is taking a walk along a road with a little girl named Andrea. They are taking a walk along a forest road, Andrea and the dwarf, the man in the white coat, whom I have not yet named. Andrea listens attentively for a few moments. Then her hand darts out and before I know it, she has snatched the carving from my hand and is sticking its head in her mouth. I am flabbergasted. I reach between the bars of the playpen and grasp the carving, now gummy with saliva. Andrea lets out a shriek and tries to pull it away. I reach the other hand through the bars and try to peel her fingers away. Like all toddlers, she has a terrific will matched by an equally terrific grip. I manage to pull the statue toward the bars and have almost extracted it—she is now gripping it in both chubby, saliva-covered fists—when she leans forward and bites my hand. I pull away, though I still have hold of the carving—we're both gripping it with determination. I reach over and grasp her wrist with my other hand. She emits her signature, ear-shattering shriek.

My mother bursts through the swinging door from the kitchen. She spots me kneeling beside the playpen, yells my name at the top of her lungs, and storms over. I realize now, although I could not have articulated it then, that she was drunk. I didn't understand "drunk" until much later. She drank, and there were always gallon bottles of scotch in the cupboard.

I let go of Andrea's wrist. Andrea drops the carving. My mother descends upon me, grabs my forearm, wrenches me to my feet. I resist, shielding my face with my free hand. I start to explain, as best I can, that Andrea was fussing and I was entertaining her—a task my two other siblings and I had made into a sort of contest because Andrea fussed a great deal—but my mother is not interested. She slaps my face and hauls me in the direction of my father's office. I know what is in store, but today, the precipitating event is unusually egregious. I glance back at Andrea, who is now standing, holding onto the bars of the playpen. Her face is an astonished blank.

My mother kicks closed the doors of the waiting room. She throws me across the room onto the couch. She pounds on me with both fists. I am crying. She has neglected to close the doors all the way, and I can hear Andrea wailing.

By itself, the beating differs little from any other beating I've received from my mother—not, in other words, meted out as logical consequences of misbehavior. She is violent when she is drunk and when she is in a rage. Her rages have become more frequent since Andrea was born.

Later that afternoon, my mother drives me to my appointment with Dr. Nemetz.

As she drives me through the rainy Boston streets on the way to Brookline—by then a daytime housekeeper has arrived to look after my siblings—my mother determines it is necessary to make sure everything in my universe continues to be internally consistent with her unique brand of logic. She informs me that I am not to say anything to Dr. Nemetz about the earlier incident.

"What about the rule?" I ask. "The no-hitting rule?"

The rule, she says grimly, has not been broken because the incident did not fall under the umbrella of occurrences to which it can be applied. She is sucking on a cigarette as she shifts the wheel-shaft gear lever, dripping ash onto the turquoise vinyl seat and the floor. The rule, she explains through cigarette-clenching lips, applies only to situations involving me and my brother. Ergo the no-hitting rule does not apply today.

It was Gloria logic. Dent-proof as fog.

I watch brick-and-limestone buildings fronting Beacon Street whiz by. The windshield wipers make uneven streaks across the glass windshield. Large drops of rain plop on the car roof. Sycamore leaves cling wetly to the windshield and the curb. The car's tires splash in and out of puddles on the rutted street.

Before I get out of the car, she extracts a promise that I will not say a word about the day's events to Dr. Nemetz.

Half an hour later, I am sitting in Dr. Nemetz's office. I sit limply in my chair across from him, looking out the window, hoping the hour will be over soon. He asks if I would like to draw today. I demur. He asks if something is wrong. I look past him to the far side of the room, where the signature couch rests on an oriental carpet disconcertingly similar to the one in my father's office. I can tell time. He has a clock on his desk. The second hand moves abysmally slowly. He addresses me. I don't answer. After a while, he leaves me alone.

Next week, next visit, same scenario. I refuse to play checkers. I won't draw. I won't do anything. He offers red lollipops—my favorite color. He suggests pickup sticks. I stare out the window at the rain.

He stands, goes to the closet, pulls out his jacket, suggests we go for a walk. He needs some tobacco. Would I like to come along? I don't care. He suggests it would probably not be good for me to wait alone in the office. I shrug. He holds out his hand. I put on my jacket, and for some reason I reach up and take his hand. We make our way down the shallow steps, out of the building, across the street, across the greenbelt in the middle of the boulevard, across the street opposite and into a tobacconist's. He chooses his tobacco. I look at the stationery in the case. He asks me if I would like something. I say no. He looks around. He points to some staplers on a shelf.

"I'll take a stapler," he says, "and a box of staples." He pays for the tobacco and the stapler and the staples. He takes the paper bag and we head out of the shop. At the curb, he takes my hand as we cross the street. Back in the office, he opens the bag, takes out the tobacco, and gives me the stapler. He shows me how to open the little hatch where the staples go and insert the staples. I spend the rest of the hour stapling pieces of paper together. He asks me what I am making.

"Books," I say.

Another week passes. Finally, exasperated, he asks me if something happened at home.

At first, I can't tell him. It is Bart Simpson's paradox a generation before Bart. Damned if I did, damned if I didn't. If I tell, I will incur my mother's wrath. But as it is now, I am not any safer than I was before the institution of the rule. What is more, now my mother believes she has me under her thumb; I am as tractable as putty in her hands. She can beat me with impunity. On the other hand, if I tell Dr. Nemetz, and he says something to my father, well, then something may change. I know my father has agreed to the rule, and I also know he believes it is being followed.

What do I have to lose?

First, I make him promise he will not call my mother. He promises. I tell him what happened. He listens intently. Then he stands up and goes to his desk. He picks up the telephone handset and dials.

"What are you doing?"

"Calling your mother. I want her to come in so I can talk to her."

I feel as though I will lose control of my sphincter. "You can't. You said you wouldn't."

"I have to."

"She'll hit me."

"No. She won't."

I sit down, stunned. Now what? The possible ramifications flow out of me in a morass of unnamed fear. I don't know what to say. I chose to tell him. Now I will face the consequences.

He reaches my mother at home, tells her to come in early to pick me up. Then he calls my father at work.

When she arrives, I am paralyzed with fear. She comes into the office, says, "Hi, sweetie," smiling excessively. Dr. Nemetz asks me to wait in the waiting room. I go out and wait. I can hear their voices dimly, but I can't tell what they are saying. I pick up a book. The waiting room is a dark, windowless, narrow little room. I think about walking downstairs, out the door, and away.

On the way home in the darkness, my mother is thin-lipped, silent, smoking ferociously. Finally, as we approach our house, she offers these words: "You'll live to regret this."

That evening, after my father comes home, my brother and Andrea are in bed, and D and I are upstairs brushing our teeth. Downstairs, there is a screaming match between my parents. High-decibel swearing. My mother, for her part, is in favor of firing Dr. Nemetz, since he is clearly not doing his job—I still make her furious, so she still has to punish me. Her violence is my fault. She does what she is being driven to do. My father is enraged that my mother cannot follow instructions given by a professional—a real psychiatrist, no less, like him. My father prevails. For me, a pyrrhic victory. No hitting.

In relatively short order, my mother figures out other means to torment me. She can control me with the threat of revelation of my ugly secret: There is no other child in my class that needs to go see a psychiatrist, she points out, is there? I am different from other children. I am poorly wrought. I am bad. The visits to the psychiatrist are to fix me. If other children were to know the truth about me, there would never be another child who would want to be my friend.

For my fifth birthday, my mother gives me a present: a little illustrated volume called *Mommies Are for Loving*. It is a picture book about a family—Mommy, Daddy, Sister, Brother, and Dog— who shower each other with love and affection in the form of hand-drawn swarms of butterfly-shaped kisses. I cannot figure out what she intends for me to make of this gift. I would rather have had a doll.

She reads the book aloud to us that same evening, sitting on the gray love seat—Andrea on her lap, Josh beside her sucking his thumb, D on a chair pretending to read a book of her own. I lean against the corner of the sofa away from the bundle of my mother and younger siblings.

"You see?" says my mother, making deliberate eye contact with me, then pointing to a picture of Mommy clutching a vacuum cleaner and smiling while Daddy plays on the floor with the dog and the brother. "This is how families are. Families love each other."

After a string of particularly frustrating sessions, I tell Chet I'm quitting. I've spent too much time and money in therapy. People act as though therapy is a substitute for life itself, I say. It isn't real life. It's fake.

I'm planning to take a self-defense course, Bay Area Model Mugging. Over a series of four-hour sessions on Sunday afternoons, women participants learn to defend themselves from physical attack using techniques borrowed from the martial arts, street fighting, and military self-defense disciplines.

A few weeks on, the Model Muggers are introduced. The Muggers are all black-belt martial artists. They are all men who are married to, partners of, coworkers with, brothers of, boyfriends or ex-boyfriends of, sons of, or widowers of women who have been molested, beaten up, raped, mugged, held captive, almost murdered, or actually murdered. They are all unpaid volunteers. Upholstered with cricket pads, goalie helmets, shoulder pads, kneepads, kidney protectors, codpieces, and sneakers wrapped in foam rubber and duct tape, the Muggers reenact violent abuse and attack situations with the participants. I have heard nothing but praise. Women who seem to have the words *victim here* tattooed like the scarlet letter onto their foreheads say the experience has been transformational.

Chet thinks the course sounds like a good idea.

Also, I've decided to find out if Dr. Nemetz is alive. If he is alive, I am going to see him. I calculate he's in his seventies.

"People have a habit of dying," I say.

Chet nods and smiles.

"I'm so glad you decided this," he says. "I was hoping someday you would. I thought about suggesting it, but my gut feeling told me it had to be your idea. I'm really glad I kept my mouth shut."

He waits. I wait.

"What will you say to him, do you think?" he asks.

"I don't know," I say. "I can't tell."

Chet nods.

"I suspect he'll find it very interesting to hear from you."

Brookline has not changed. I take the streetcar, which creaks down the same set of tracks on Beacon Street. The same row of brick-and-stone buildings. The same carved lion's head keystone above the arched doorway at 1419 Beacon Street.

Dr. Nemetz tells me he recognizes me. He looks the same, except he's an old man. His office is the same, the carpet is the same, but the toy cupboard is gone. He says he would have a hard time these days getting onto the floor to play with little kids.

I ask Dr. Nemetz if he remembers the fateful afternoon when I called bullshit on my mother. The Gorgon Medusa in a world where there was no Perseus. When he betrayed me to my abusers. Which I'd been paying for ever since.

He tells me he doesn't remember the incident, exactly, although he does remember having several conversations with my mother. He remembers that my parents represented me as a child who was out of control. I listen in horror as he tells me how they characterized me: an unnatural child, a monster. He tells me how they maintained they feared I would harm my brother, who was little and helpless and without guile. He says he did not know, really, about the violence, other than what my parents—especially my mother—told him.

"How could you not have known when I told you about it myself?" I ask. "Right here. When I was four years old."

He opens his mouth. He closes it. He reminds me for a moment of a guppy in a fish tank, their little round mouths that open and close, open and close, silently, eyes bulging in unblinking stares.

"I . . ." he says. He stops. He looks at me blankly.

Dr. Nemetz used to play games with his face to make me laugh when I was upset. He'd stick out his tongue, then pull on one ear so his tongue rolled to one side of his mouth, then pull the other ear to make his tongue roll the other way. Then he'd pull the skin below his Adam's apple. Then his tongue would disappear with a little "gulp" as his mouth snapped shut. I'd always laugh. Stupid, I know, but some gags just work with little kids; no matter how upset they are, you can make them howl with laughter if you use the right trick. Try tearing up a piece of paper for a cranky ten-month-old sometime.

But the cute tongue-swallowing act isn't going to do it for me in my thirties. Fortunately, he doesn't try it. He shakes his head.

"What would you have wanted me to do?"

"Get me out of there. Put me into foster care. Let me come live with you."

"I could not have done that, even if I had wanted it."

He raises his hands, momentarily, palms up, in a gesture of helplessness.

For a moment, I am transported back to Miami Beach three decades before. A gust of wind over the breakers. A little girl stands watching a red-and-yellow beach ball beyond her reach. She watches the waves carry her ball away, outward, ever outward, until it disappears into a blue and indifferent sea.

I pick up my coat. I've decided the hour is over. Politely and icily, I pull my checkbook out of my purse and ask him how much he wants to be paid.

He shakes his head, no, no. Don't be ridiculous, he says, it was his pleasure. He asks if we should talk again. I say I do not know. I say I'll write him a letter.

I make it out the door. I rush down the two flights of stairs, and by the time I reach the ground floor, I am convulsed by tears of rage. A friend of longstanding who lives in Connecticut has offered to meet me and is waiting for me in her car in front of the building. I get in and cry, unable to control myself. Whether I've ever admitted to their existence or not, my feelings now own me outright.

My friend hugs me and then starts the car. We pull away from the curb into the twilight, the usual late-winter New England gloom, lit only by the soggy glow of streetlamps. We drive toward Boston, where we will stay with her brother for the night. We stop at a stoplight across from the Charles River. The light in the gloaming softens as clouds part. Night capitulates to day for a moment before the sun disappears. The term in France where I lived for eight years is *le soleil se couche*—the sun puts itself to bed, as though someone comes to tuck it in. I can see the river in front of us—gray and flat and motionless. Then, beside me, the car door opens. A little girl with a mop of blonde curls stands there. She is about four years old. Wordlessly, she climbs into the car, onto my seat. I move toward the hand brake a little bit to make room, but she does not seem to need any extra space. She seems to have brought space with her. My friend, who is driving, watches the road. She appears not to notice the arrival of this second passenger. I do not call her attention to this pixie revenant, the child—I realize some years later—I myself annihilated in a desperate wish for my mother's love.

Back in California a few days later, I go to see Chet. He asks how the session went. I describe it to him. He asks me if I was upset by Dr. Nemetz's indifference to what was happening at home. He asks if I was angry that he betrayed me to my mother.

"Yes," I say. I bite my lips. I turn away. I am still unable to cry in front of him.

Then I tell him about the little girl who got into the car at the stoplight.

He listens. Then he nods. I wait, watching for some clue to his reaction. I am terrified he will judge me.

"You think I'm crazy, don't you? A little girl only I can see gets into a car at a stoplight and never gets out." I'm preparing to do the only thing I know how to do: leap up and flee.

"Where is she now?"

"Well, let's put it this way," I say. "She hasn't gone anywhere."

Chet touches his fingers together; he looks at me.

"I don't think you're crazy," he says. Then he asks, "Were you near water, when that happened?"

"Yes," I say. "Right across from the river. At a stoplight. About to cross the bridge. How did you know?"

He looks at me, looks at his hands, reflectively.

"I don't know, really," he says. "It's just that those kinds of experiences, when they happen, people are usually near a body of water."

Chet, in not once suggesting my perceptions were wrong, did something no other therapist I'd met had ever done before. He accepted and affirmed my feelings and my perceptions. He did not insist what was happening was really something else. By not insisting the material world was all that mattered, he validated something I'd always hoped was true: I did not have to be enslaved by what other people said or thought or did.

I've come to understand since then that those who insist on life being entirely literal perform an act of co-optation. By insisting there is nothing other than what they themselves can see and have seen—never mind anyone else—such persons force everyone else to submit to a kind of nihilistic materialism.

My father was one of these, ridiculing the mere idea of an afterlife, mocking the possibility of extraterrestrial beings living in some form on other planets. Life itself was not important, other than his own.

For despots—authoritarian leaders like Vladimir Putin or Donald Trump—this conviction is the very basis of their self-aggrandizing narcissism. If the truth lies outside of us, it is in someone else's hands. Then, whatever ails us emotionally or spiritually can be cured only by someone or something who is not the person herself. As soon as we need that pill to feel better, that glass of wine at the end of the day, we are robbed of our agency. To feel complete, we must submit to the authority of a person or a government or a medication that will keep us whole. This state is a state of annihilation, where we have no connection to our own interiors, our spiritual space, wherein a true understanding of connection with the universe and with other life-forms—people, animals, fish, trees, microorganisms, extraterrestrials—begins.

In an interview in *The Journal of Transpersonal Psychology*, Dr. Stanislav Grof, a Czech-born psychiatrist, founder of the modern transpersonal movement and, during the 1960s and 1970s, principal researcher at the Maryland Psychiatric Research Center, where he was the principal investigator exploring the therapeutic potential of psychedelic drugs, described the significance of the transpersonal perspective:

> As a culture, we are paying a great toll for having lost spirituality and oriented ourselves completely towards the external world. This has led to a destructive and self-destructive way of being in the world in which we are a threat to future life on the planet. So bringing in a psychology that not only recognizes spirituality, but one that also has technologies where people can actually have spiritual experiences, is extremely beneficial for people individually as well as for humanity collectively.[3]

During the winter of 2020, I was in New York for a few months, a trip foreshortened because I'd had to rush back to France on orders of the French government because of the arrival of COVID-19 and the international pandemonium that ensued.

I was leaving the subway platform at the 125th Street and Lexington Avenue station, headed out through the turnstile, when a scream rose behind me, a cry so bloodcurdling I was certain someone was being killed. I whirled around. The train doors closed, and the train clanked forward out of the station. A chunky girl of about thirteen or fourteen in a pink T-shirt, with a pink rucksack, ran frantically alongside the moving train, braids bouncing. She gestured wildly. Red-faced, gasping, she pounded on the subway's doors and windows, screaming through tears. Beside me, another woman on her way out of the station paused and shook her head. The girl's shrieks boomed off the white tile of the domed tunnel.

"Someone's under the train. Someone got killed," said the woman. She reached out and clutched my shoulder.

"Maybe a toddler," I said, my blood running cold. "Maybe her sister." We moved closer to one another, preparing instinctively for a view of gore. More people gathered. Beyond the barrier, another girl, a friend or classmate, ran up beside her, talking, gesturing.

"Stop the fucking train!" someone shouted. "The kid's going to have a heart attack."

Then a man ran alongside the train, waving at the conductor's mirror. "Stop the train. Someone's hurt!"

The train lurched to a halt.

The conductor leaned out his window, then opened his door. "What? What is it?"

The girl shook and shuddered and hiccupped. She turned then and ran opposite the direction of motion toward the car she'd exited. She pounded on the door.

Gasping, the friend shouted to the conductor. "It was her phone. She forgot her phone."

"Jesus Christ," said the woman beside me, wilting. "What in the—I was about to call 911."

The door to the carriage opened. The girl ran in and retrieved her phone. She emerged hiccupping. People began to disperse, shaking their heads.

If I'd been anywhere near her, my inner schoolmarm may have loosed herself. I confess to feeling something more akin to vexation than sympathy toward this girl. How could she become so unglued over a phone? Had she had an upbringing that had produced not one iota of resourcefulness? She apparently did not have a clue how to function without being plugged in. The moment she lost her phone, she lost it. I'm not talking about just the phone, but *it*, her mind, her life, and her spiritual wholeness. It was like watching someone melt away, or become suddenly unmoored in space, out of touch, out of control, powerless, furious, and terrified. Because of a mobile phone.

I try to imagine this poor girl riding a bike home from a friend's house and getting a flat tire a mile from her mother's house. What would she do then? Or perhaps I am completely out of touch.

Perhaps kids don't ride bikes to one another's houses anymore. Or their friends live no more than a block away.

I've found myself returning mentally to the scene again and again. Was it about connectedness? Was it about not being able to call her mother? Her friend must have had at least some of the contacts on her own phone. I don't think connection was the problem. Her reaction was about something else: about living in a world in which all of life—her life, at least—had become in its own way so devoid of situations for which she could not access an answer instantaneously, she could not for a moment figure out what to do when there was a slight warp in the road. The solution to every conceivable doubt, question, and conundrum her life presented was always in her hand. She had no internal resources. All the tendrils holding her to existence were found on her phone and nowhere else. She was terrified of autonomy. If I were to push this image to its limit, I would come up with a version of *The Matrix*, where humans are yoked, mind and body, in service of a computer that has constructed a false reality to deceive them.[4]

Under our version of authoritarianism in the twenty-first century, we as witless consumers don't even need the government to oppress us. The joke is on us: We're all working for the man. We're doing it to ourselves. We're complicit in our own unraveling.

Chapter 3

BREAKING BAD AT HARVARD

There is a photograph taken in the early 1960s of me as a child of four or five that I can't now lay my hands on.

I am seated on a black wool mid-century-modern ottoman in front of the fireplace in my parents' suburban Boston living room on a winter afternoon. I'm dressed in a plaid brown-and-green dress. Puffed sleeves with tight, white, unforgiving cuffs clasp the flesh of my upper arms like admonitory fingers. Little bars of plaid fabric are stitched across my chest. My hands clutch the carved wooden handles at either side of the seat. My hair is brushed hastily over to one side, held with a barrette. I was dressed and primped hurriedly for this occasion, late one afternoon. It is the afternoon following a very bad night, during which I'd been beaten, and a subsequent morning spent locked in my father's waiting room.

My parents, who both presided over the photo session, demanded I let go of the seat and put my hands in my lap. My father must have repeated the injunction a number of times before giving up and snapping the photo anyway. There was a pressing reason for their needing to take it just then, that afternoon—not one of those afternoons when all four of us were being photographed together. Just me. Alone. In the living room, for a designated purpose other than a faked artifact of a happy childhood.

What disturbed me about the photograph was not the dourness of the dress or the hair, or the white backs of my hands clenching the handles of the ottoman or the barrette or the fact I had to sit that afternoon for a photo without my siblings. It was the blank rivet of my eyes on somewhere, themselves revealing nothing. When I first came across the photo, it appeared fuzzy, as though out of focus, as though unsteady hands had snapped the shutter.

Not so, I realize. My eyes are frozen into a look I now recognize as dissociation. I can't look into the lens because I can't look at my parents, these people so bent on my annihilation.

I discovered that day I could avert my eyes toward an unseeable elsewhere, and with that I learned to perfect the thousand-yard stare into the place no one else could touch. That day was the day I annihilated myself to survive.

When I was in my twenties, I destroyed most of the photographs I had of myself as a child, as though in destroying them I could remake myself into someone else: someone who came from a family who loved her. I suspect, in my heart of hearts, that photo was among them. The photo, I learned later, was a mug shot for the psychiatrists my parents spent part of the day contacting. At least one had asked my parents for a photo prior to agreeing to meet with me. Racial profiling? Judgment before the fact? The burden of the family insanity was mine to bear. I was to be sent to the shrinks to figure out if I could be altered, like a poorly fitting skin suit, into some more malleable and better child, different from the one my parents got. If, and only if, the shrinks succeeded, my parents would then be able to stop beating me.

My parents were both proud bearers of recently minted Harvard (in my mother's case Radcliffe) degrees. My father had completed training at Harvard Medical School and was employed as a psychiatric resident at a Harvard-affiliated hospital.

Looking back, I see my parents as an embodiment of the trajectory of modern academic medicine, especially psychiatry.

Success in this world is about the ability to manipulate, transact, and gaslight. Every skill and attribute necessary to secure one's seat in this reputation-gilding, money-making machine is antithetical to the primary tenets of the Hippocratic oath: to relieve suffering and to do no harm. Being part of it means one's life path rolls out like a carpet strewn with lilies. A mediocre man by any measure, my father especially excelled because he mastered the most central skill of modern psychiatry: persuading subjects there was something wrong with them, while there was no fault to be found with those who did them harm.

My mother, for her part, earned her PhD under the tutelage of Dr. Henry A. Murray, whose clinical experiment, "Studies of Stressful Interpersonal Disputations," was implicated in the breakdown and subsequent psychopathology of Theodore Kaczynski, who later became known as the Unabomber.

My parents personified the stereotype of those who are drawn to these lines of work: They harbor deep-seated, unacknowledged mental illness. My mother, for instance, was an unacknowledged alcoholic, like her own father. I believe she was beaten as a child, although she did not talk about it. I've described my mother to some therapists, when pushed for an explanation of her actions, as likely suffering from a psychological form of Munchausen syndrome by proxy.[1] I now believe she suffered from borderline personality disorder, perfectly matched with my father's malignant narcissism. My parents' personalities were a textbook combination, fitting together like lock and key. Where there's a malignant narcissist, there's inevitably a borderline not far behind.

As for my father, pedophilia formed the backbone of his genealogy. His family on his mother's side was filthy with it. Neither wealthy nor particularly gifted at anything nor likeable enough for the real corridors of power, my father eventually became an academic psychiatrist, padding his income with consulting work at state mental hospitals. An alcoholic and medical drug addict, he was incapable of holding on to money. Like all cons, he was nothing if not susceptible to other cons. He was drawn to those with money or who he believed had more social status. His dentist found him useful for investment schemes that always ultimately went belly-up. A uranium claim. A gold mine.

While the primary draw of the mind-scrubbing fields may for any individual initially be well-intentioned, as often happens, a few years on with initiates in these fields, ego dynamics take over. Even if the supplicant isn't a malignant narcissist, becoming a Harvard psychiatrist or medical doctor is an ego-inflating, grandiosity-fluffing mega-drug in its own right. Nothing is wrong with Harvard psychiatrists or Harvard intellectuals by definition. They are as close to God on earth as the intelligentsia get.

Try telling one he (or she) is wrong about something to his (or her) face—with documentation—if you care to test this hypothesis. They're not a humble lot.

My mother had no moral compass and simply did and said what my father expected, except when her own psychoses became so acute her alcohol-infused rages were her best and only go-to. I was chosen as the living object onto whom my parents could comfortably project their rage, anger, and hatred. Compassion did not exist for them, any more than it existed for Henry A. Murray. The real point is to destroy the visionary and the vision, the person or child in a family or institution or culture who either wittingly or unwittingly embodies the truth about what is terribly horribly wrong. To preserve the accepted lie, this person has to die.

By the time I was in my later childhood, I may as well have been dead. I ceased to feel. My emotions lived in another world. The only protection I had from my parents was to leave my body, to leave my mind, and take up residence in the lonely elsewhere of traumatic dissociation. I did not begin to figure out what had happened to me until I was in my twenties. And that revelation came at a terrible price.

My parents were educated and employed at Harvard during one of the most promising times in recent history, when, momentarily, the explorations of a few individuals into spirituality and mental health were poised to make the twentieth century a century of human progress. While the intellectual cauldron around them boiled over and Beat culture embodied in the visions of Jack Kerouac and Allen Ginsberg upset the silver tea services of a tweedy, upper-crust, post–World War II academic establishment, my parents lived in their own *folie à deux*, in perfect sync with the rigid class structure governed by the social institutions of the day. My parents' single-minded occupation was not being found out as the imposters they were.

During these years, two original research projects were hatched at their hallowed alma mater: one a study in behavioral psychology, the other a study in mysticism and spirituality. Between them, these two experiments and their aftermath have limned the field of "psychology" as we now know it. They were designed and executed by two very different men under the broad academic umbrellas of the Department of Social Relations and the Department of Philosophy.

"Studies of Stressful Interpersonal Disputations"—hereafter referred to as Murray's experiment—was the brainchild of my mother's major professor, Harvard University Professor of Clinical Psychology Dr. Henry A. Murray, known as the father of personality theory. The experiment, completed in 1962, was a final variation on a long-term investigation into personality that Murray had commenced in the mid-1940s, the "Multiform Assessments of Personality Development Among Gifted College Men."

The second Harvard experiment, "Drugs and Mysticism: An Analysis of the Relationship Between Psychedelic Drugs and the Mystical State of Consciousness," was designed by Walter N. Pahnke for his PhD thesis project under the supervision of Dr. Timothy Leary, who, in 1962, was a lecturer and clinical psychologist at Harvard, as part of the Harvard Psilocybin Project.

The experiments could not have been more different in concept, scope, or outcome. The manner in which their results were eventually received both at Harvard and in the broader world defined how psychology and psychotherapy evolved both in theory and in practice in the United States for the next fifty years.

Murray was born in 1893 in New York. A true New York society blue blood by birth, Murray trained first as a physician at Columbia University and went on to study biochemistry at Cambridge University. After completing a surgical internship, Murray took a career-defining detour in 1923, when he read Swiss psychoanalyst C. G. Jung's seminal book, *Psychological Types*. The book, it appears, affirmed his feelings about his own interests. Years later, he recalled he had spent more time "than was considered proper for a surgeon seeking psychogenic factors in my patients."[2]

Murray has been characterized by those who knew him as "brilliant and complex." His peers, research associates, and colleagues also described him, by turns, as patronizing and narcissistic, as well as privileged and autocratic. He was the model of the entitled "establishment" male. Psychologist David Ricks, one of five coinvestigators conducting Murray's experiment, said of Murray, "He used to talk about GI culture and hatred of officers among enlisted men. It showed our comparative status in his eyes."[3] He recalled a sense of relief in 1960, when he finally broke away from Murray's lab, comparing Murray's intrusiveness and presumption of closeness to that of someone who behaved toward the members of the lab like a father toward sons.

"I resented the assumed closeness, and I hated the praise, which seemed manipulative and condescending," Ricks said.[4]

Murray dedicated the latter part of his career to reenvisioning academic psychology, which had been devoted for decades to the systematic study of behavioral patterns of individuals. Academic psychologists, he declared, had turned the study of human behavior into something resembling theoretical physics. In his view, their research had little if anything to do with actual humans. His goal was to liberate the field from this ossified pursuit and to transform it into an integrated science, which encompassed the study of the conscious and the unconscious mind, as well as individual needs, drives, and motivations. He coined a neologism, *personology*, to describe his new science of personality.

Despite Murray's not-so-private belief that he was an upstart, an embattled soul fighting against the intellectual machine at Harvard, he was anything but. He was, rather, a grandiose intellectual dilettante who envied the talents of the truly creative.[5] Murray was an aficionado of the author Herman Melville, even writing an unpublished biography of Melville, for whom he'd developed an admiration, one that bordered on fetish. The poet Conrad Aiken, a close Murray friend, read the first few chapters of this opus at Murray's request. Then, during Thanksgiving dinner at the Murray household in November 1939, he denounced it incisively.

The work was astoundingly bad.

"You think you've baleened, but in fact you've ballooned," jeered Aiken.[6] When asked to elaborate, a drunken Aiken described the manuscript to Murray as "inflated and overblown" and "a piece of gigantism." The work placed Murray's narcissism and grandiosity squarely on display.

Unlike most American academic psychologists of his time, Murray was smitten with Jung's work, especially Jung's theories of the collective unconscious and his writing about universal archetypes. Murray had spent the better part of the spring of 1925 with Jung in Zurich, meeting with him for hours every day and on weekends, sailing Lake Zurich on Jung's boat. He described Sigmund Freud as "a strange genius who made some of the shrewdest guesses," and he mocked Freud's academic heirs as insufferable, untrained idiots, who, having never been schooled in the basic sciences, spent their time engaged in metaphysical mind games and "polymorphous perversities of logic."[7]

By the late 1950s, Murray's ideas about human nature had evolved from the purely analytical. He theorized there was no better way of mapping the true character of the human personality than through studying interpersonal relationships. Rather than view a person in isolation—as behaviorists tended to do—Murray now wanted to study the human being through what he considered the most basic, elemental human relationship, the smallest social unit, a pair of two people, which he called "the dyad."

Murray initiated his "Studies of Stressful Interpersonal Relations" in 1957, shortly before he retired. That year, he recruited a group of "23 comprehensively assessed college sophomores, and then, in a more refined way, in 1960 a comparable aggregate of 21 subjects."[8]

Prior to agreeing to participate, students were given no information about the experiment. Instead, they were asked to state a positive answer to the question "Would you be willing to work at the Psychological Clinic Annex (48 Mt. Auburn St.) (at current Harvard rate) helping our researches by taking a series of tests through the academic year?"[9]

As in the previous "Multiform Assessments of Personality Development" studies, the experiment was designed to gather as much personal and biographical information from each subject as possible. Psychological assessment included the Thematic Apperception Test (TAT), which Murray developed during the 1930s in collaboration with his long-time mistress, Jungian analyst Christiana Morgan. The TAT employs a set of thirty-one ambiguous pictures shown to subjects in sequence. The images range from the merely peculiar to the truly weird. In one picture, a young woman holding a book stands in the foreground in front of a plowed field. A laborer and a plow horse figure in the background, while an evidently pregnant woman stands to one side. In another, a man bends over the figure of a sleeping woman with his hand raised above her forehead. Participants are asked to create a story about what was taking place in each one. The TAT was designed, according to its creators, to explore personality and reveal internal conflicts, drives, and motivations. The ambiguous images inspired the subject to express their beliefs and feelings through narrative. This, posited Murray, gave experimenters an assortment of meta personal snippets Murray considered a good basis for personality assessment.

The subjects were also given the Rorschach inkblot test and asked to submit an essay about their "personal philosophy of life."

Although based on a similar series of tests and interviews, Murray's experiment differed from the earlier "Multiform Assessments of Personality Development" in a key way. These new studies purposefully elicited strong emotional responses. The encounters with research staff were stage-managed to provoke anger and anxiety among the participants by exposing them to aggressive questioning from graduate students who were playacting as lawyers. Following submission of the personal-philosophy essay, the research staff staged a discussion of the subject's work.

"At this point, you are introduced to the young lawyer and in his company escorted to the brilliantly lighted room where the debate will take place in front of a one-way mirror," wrote Murray in a 1963 article in *American Psychologist*.[10] Once the participant was hooked up to a cardiotachometer, the interaction between subject and lawyer commenced. After a few minutes of ordinary conversation, "the lawyer's criticism becomes far more vehement, sweeping, and personally abusive than you were led to expect."[11] The point of the exercise was to anger the participant by dressing him down and deriding the quality of his essay.

Throughout the experiment, the subject's heart and respiratory rate were recorded. A video record was made of the entire encounter, which subjects were required to view during follow-up interviews.

"You will see yourself making numerous grimaces and gestures of which you were unconscious at the time, and you will hear yourself uttering incongruent, disjunctive, and unfinished sentences,"

Murray wrote. "You are likely to be somewhat shocked by your performance and will be moved to identify with yourself as you were feeling and thinking during those stressful moments."

Although Murray's stated goal throughout was "to construct a coherent formulation of each personality," the experiments themselves humiliated the subjects in what was little more than a tactical enterprise to shatter the subject's sense of emotional unity. I concluded, many years on, my parents had learned how to flay me emotionally by way of Murray's example.

Murray's scheme was devoid of any consideration for the student volunteers. The experience, according to many, was brutal. Many emerged either in a state of rage or overcome by feelings of defenselessness.

One subject—code-named "Cringle"—gave the following account of his experience: "We were led into the room with bright lights, very bright. [I] had a sensation somewhat akin to someone being strapped on the electric chair with these electrodes . . . [I was] getting hotter and more irritated and my heartbeat going up . . . and sweating terribly . . ."[12]

Another subject, code-named "Trump," described his experience with the interrogator: "[Dr. G] . . . came waltzing over and he put on those electrodes . . . And then [Mr. R] . . . who was bubbling over, dancing around, started to talk to me about [how] he liked my suit . . . ." The subject described becoming so enraged during the course of the interrogation he was inclined to move the encounter outside so that he could confront the interrogators mano a mano. He would have done so, he recalled, save for the electrodes attached to his body that stopped him.[13]

What Murray intended to do with the data he gathered or why he felt they were of value was unclear. As Murray wrote in *American Psychologist, "cui bono"*—for what use?

As they stand, they are nothing but raw data, meaningless as such. The question is, "What meaning, what intellectual news, can be extracted from them?"

The emotional evisceration of his study subjects in service of recording a fabricated scenario of psychological torture meted out upon unsuspecting undergraduates was of more than passing interest to Murray. Murray's real interest lay in gauging, assessing, and manipulating power relationships.

During the Second World War, in 1943, Murray had become a defense intelligence consultant in Washington at the Office of Strategic Services, the precursor to today's CIA. His mission was to assess prospective intelligence agents for field preparedness. Recruits underwent a grueling series of personality tests lasting three and a half days. They were subjected to high-pressure interviews by seven senior staff members, including psychiatrists, psychologists, sociologists, and seven junior staff, most of whom were graduate students in psychology.

"It was all very good fun," Murray said of his OSS experience, "terrifically interesting, terrific fun."[14]

He described his time in 1945 in China, where he evaluated Chinese paratroopers for intelligence operations behind Japanese lines, in similar terms.

"I enjoyed myself hugely in China." Murray, it seemed, experienced the war as a kind of *Bill & Ted's Excellent Adventure*, a goofy reprieve from business as usual at Harvard.

But business as usual captained by Murray would be implicated in some dire events.

Theodore Kaczynski was fifteen years old when he arrived at Harvard as a freshman. He was seventeen when he was recruited as a junior into Murray's experiment. To describe him as "naive" or "vulnerable" does not do him justice.

After Harvard, Kaczynski, who was a gifted mathematician, embarked on a successful academic career but abandoned it within ten years. By 1971, Kaczynski was living a survivalist's existence in a cabin outside Lincoln, Montana, shunning all technological and mechanical conveniences, including electric light and indoor plumbing. His practice of sabotaging building and road development in the forest near his cabin evolved by 1978 into bomb making. Many of his devices were delivered through the mail. All of them were directed at powerful men, most of them scientists who, Kaczynski felt, were contributing to the destruction of the natural world. Kaczynski was eventually arrested in 1996 after his brother provided the FBI with leads based on personal letters that linked the bomber to his manifesto. Controversy raged for a time over an article and then a book written by former philosophy professor Alston Chase that implied that Murray's experiment contributed to Kaczynski's feelings of alienation and betrayal at Harvard and was responsible for the pathology that caused him to start blowing up academic scientists.[15]

Many mental health professionals asserted Kaczynski's pathology could not be attributed to Murray's experiment and insisted his pathology was an instance of correlation rather than causation. They were wrong. They were engaging in the activity 99 percent of mental health professionals engage in when confronted with the fact of abuse among their professional kin: They deny, they gaslight, they close ranks. Kaczynski's participation in Murray's experiment was no accident. His recruitment into the study was calculated. Research protocols directed screeners to cherry-pick young men like Kaczynski who already felt alienated and intimidated at Harvard.

According to the study description, "Volunteers were selected from among those students enrolled in a large social relations course who scored either high or low on scales assessing alienation."[16] The goal was to solicit young men at either end of an extreme for this particular personality trait. Anecdotal reporting indicated those who tested as "less alienated" had very different responses to the experiment from those who tested as "extremely alienated."[17] Kaczynski tested as extremely alienated. Stressed to his limits during the experiment, seventeen-year-old Kaczynski went off the rails. He and the other young men were not offered any therapeutic assistance that might have helped them process what happened during the experiment. Kaczynski grew into a bitter, alienated man who sought revenge.

There was another creepy synchronicity between my mother, Murray's experiment, and Kaczynski.

My mother was born and raised in Lombard, Illinois, a half hour west of Chicago, Ted Kaczynski's hometown. She was born in 1925. Kaczynski was born in 1942. Scientific positivism would dictate I ascribe their shared childhood locale to mere coincidence. An accident of statistics.

I no longer believe this.

As I've gotten older and wiser and more familiar with the patterns of transpersonal relationships in my own life and those I've observed in lives of others, I see very little in the way of mere coincidence, particularly when one considers the frequency with which these events occur. I offer another example: My parents had three very close friends—rather the men were my father's close friends, which meant we spent inordinate amounts of time with their families. Thanksgiving. Passover. Summer holidays. Each couple had a daughter who died or was killed in young adulthood: one of ovarian cancer, one hit by a bus, and one in the World Trade Center on 9/11. My own younger sister Andrea died in her forties of metastatic colon cancer, which had gone undetected until she was terminally ill.

Andrea was a slight and frail-looking child until her eighth year, when she was molested by my father's young uncle, Eddie, my grandmother's youngest brother. He entrapped her in a downstairs bathroom while guests at my elder sister's bat mitzvah party were frolicking upstairs. Soon after, she refused to allow her hair to be washed or cut. She would not permit anyone but my mother to touch her. She would not respond to or countenance my father. Her table manners became disgusting. Sitting across from her at the family table, regarding her as she grasped slippery haunches of barbecue chicken and shoved them into her mouth, head bent possessively over her plate to evade my father's advances—he habitually walked around the table and snatched food from our plates when it suited him—I could not eat. My response to the dynamics around food in my parents' house was to stop eating.

By the time I was fourteen, I was an obsessive dieter. By fifteen, I refused to eat meals at the family table altogether. Andrea's response was to keep eating. And eating and eating and eating. By her early teens, she could not fit into regular girls' clothing. By the time she was in graduate school, she was morbidly obese.

Eddie, the molester, my father's young uncle, was a mere five years his senior. Eddie came from a line of sexual predators, all hailing from the same side of the family, the Russian Jewish side, the Berman side, my father's mother's clan. Eddie also molested his own daughter, Linda, a fact I deduced after attending her wedding ceremony in Los Angeles in my teens, a spectacle of freakish pageantry: The back wall of the sanctuary retracted into the ceiling to reveal the spotlight-illuminated bride, who then walked down a white carpet on her father's arm toward her new man. A real Barbie Princess Bride performance. A few hours after the ceremony, shortly after the bride and groom had departed ostensibly for their honeymoon, she fled from him, offering no explanation. My grandmother managed to obtain his phone number from Linda's distraught mother. Courteous and patient— not a bad guy at all, really, from the way it sounded—he said, "There was no communication." He refused to say anything more. The marriage was annulled.

Two of my father's cousins were molested by other Berman uncles, Eddie's elder brothers. Mary Etta, a cousin who lived in San Jose where she worked as a computer programmer, who often babysat for us, was one of them.

Years later, when I was in college, I visited her in San Francisco, where she was taking premed courses. She had quit her programming job and was planning to attend medical school. She'd made the mistake of telling my father about what had happened to her at the hands of one of the uncles. Foolishly, she thought being a psychiatrist, he would take her part. My father told her she was confabulating.

I remember regarding her speechlessly, staring at her wedge-shaped face, framed by brown hair in her dark living room, located in the upstairs of a house owned by an elderly woman. Mary Etta told me she wanted to become a psychiatrist to help other women who had undergone the same kind of violation she had. She knew, she said, there were others in the family who had endured similar abuse. I told her about what had happened to Andrea at D's bat mitzvah. She'd been there. She and her boyfriend had stayed with my siblings and me for several days afterward, while my parents went away. I asked if she had known, if anyone had told her. She said no.

"Did your parents know?" asked Mary Etta then, lighting a cigarette. "Any of you tell them?"

"Andrea didn't want us to tell. D may have told. I don't know what they knew," I said.

"Don't know what they knew," echoed Mary Etta, looking away. "No one knows what they knew."

A few months later, Mary Etta departed California for Michigan, where she'd grown up, to move in with her divorced sister and help care for her sister's children while she attended medical school. My parents never heard from her again. After repeated phone calls to a purported forwarding number, my mother commenced a familiar smear campaign. History was rewritten, true to family tradition. She was a confabulator, a troubled woman who could not commit. She'd broken off two engagements, decisions certainly meriting condemnation. She had strange values. Moving in with her divorced sister while trying to get a medical education at the same time? Ridiculous. But the real problem was Mary Etta's rejection of my parents. Anyone who snubbed my parents was deemed deeply defective. Mary Etta had done the deed.

Mary Etta's first cousin, Rana, also described as "a weird one," was another of my father's second cousins. She was married to a character named Ike.

Ike was a lumbering, fat, ugly man. His face was as pock-marked as a lava field. He wore a goatee. He reeked of cheap aftershave, bourbon, and stale cigarette smoke. He worked in a business no one discussed.

In the early sixties, when D and I were little and still living in Massachusetts, Ike exposed himself to us. Rana and Ike and their children always attended the endlessly long family *seders.* D and I would be put to bed in a room we shared along with Rana and Ike's daughter, Michelle, who was a few years our junior. She slept on a cot. Later in the evening, while the other adults were downstairs visiting, Ike would enter our room. Although Michelle was his intended target—even in the dark we could see he was doing something to her—he often exposed himself to us. He'd go to her bed, open his fly, and take out his penis. She'd take it obediently in her hand and put it into her mouth. He'd taught her to suck him off. We'd pull our blankets over our heads. Eventually, D and I developed a sort of perverted game out of the experience. We gave "Ike's penis" a persona of its own. He'd go on trips, go to work, take children to school. A twisted little girls' game to defuse the horror of what we were seeing.

One Passover night, shortly after he'd closed the door behind him, we heard a commotion on the stairs. Rana burst into the room, in extreme distress, her mother at her heels.

"Where's Ike?" Rana shouted. "Is Ike in here? Was Ike in here?"

"Hush, Rana," her mother said, grabbing her arm. "Ike left an hour ago. What would he be doing here? You'll wake the children." She hustled Rana out of the room. Ike must have feigned a departure through my father's office waiting room, out the back door, offering some excuse about having parked the car up the street. Closer to leave out the back, right? Rather than departing, he'd come up the stairs, which, conveniently, were out of the view of those in the dining room. Once he'd finished, he must have left surreptitiously out the waiting-room door.

A few days later, the Leiderman tribunal—my mother, my

grandmother, my father—had a go at Rana. Rana, declared my grandmother, had always been a weird little girl. Nothing like her sister, Risa. Risa the perfect daughter, married to a rabbi.

My grandfather never participated in this activity or the general pattern of the family psychopathy. He was the single member of the extended family who showed me any kindness. During the summers when they stayed with us, when I was between the ages of three and six, my grandfather would meet me when I got off the summer-camp bus at the corner of our street and walk me home, holding my hand.

My grandfather was born in 1894 in England, where his Ukrainian parents had stopped for a few years to obtain visas for the United States during their flight from Kyiv. His nature was entirely unlike that of my grandmother and her family.

Ike eventually went to prison—not for child molestation but for some unrelated criminal activity, about which I was ignorant.

One night, years later, I learned that Rana, too, had been molested as a child by one of the Berman uncles. I was at a boyfriend's house, and there, suddenly, a late-night public service announcement for a local television station revealed Rana, hair uncoiffed, wearing not the pastel-and-white suburban garb of years past but a midi skirt, sandals, a fringed shawl, recounting what had happened to her and her children. She was living in Berkeley and hadn't spoken to her parents since she'd left her marriage and her family of origin years before. She was involved with a collective for women like herself. She'd left Ike when she realized the man she had married was molesting her children, a pattern, she said, often repeated by women who had been themselves molested as children.

A few years later, after I'd cut off ties with my own family of origin, I tried to contact her. I called and left her a message. Rana never returned my call. Rana did exactly what I would have done and what Mary Etta had done: made sure no one in the family knew where she was or what she was doing.

What are the odds of four terribly close, privileged, well-heeled, well-educated friends all losing a child to accident, *force majeure*, or a disease that went undiagnosed until it was way too late? My father and his dear friends were men of loose morals, of lascivious appetites, of execrable personal boundaries. Were these friendships mere coincidence? Or just a matter of birds of a feather flocking together? The eldest son of one of them raped a little girl when he was in his teens. He was never prosecuted. The father paid off the girl's family. How do I know this? Because I listened. I listened to the father brag unashamedly about it at my father's sixtieth birthday party. What a man his son was, what a specimen of masculinity, taking out his *schmeckel* at the age of fourteen and doing it. This son, unsurprisingly, became my father's lifelong lawyer and the trustee of his estate. His sister, one of the dead daughters of my father's good friends, was killed in the attack on the World Trade Center on 9/11.

Alden Wessman, a former research associate of Murray who has long been bothered by the unethical dimension of Murray's experiment, told Alston Chase in an interview, "Later, I thought we took and took and used them and what did we give them in return?"[18]

Years on, subjects still recalled the experience with horror.

In 1987, in a follow-up interview, Cringle, one of the study subjects, recalled the "anger and embarrassment . . . the glass partition . . . the electrodes and wires running up our sleeves."

Drill, another participant, still had "very vivid general memories of the experience. . . . I remember someone putting electrodes and a blood pressure counter on my arm just before the filming . . . [I] was startled by [my interlocutor's] venom . . . I remember responding with unabating rage."

Locust wrote, "I remember appearing one afternoon for a 'debate' and being hooked up to electrodes and sat in a chair with bright lights and being told a movie was being made . . . I remember being shocked by the severity of the attack, and I remember feeling helpless to respond."[19]

What were the consequences, for Murray, of executing a social relations experiment wherein the study subjects were treated as artifacts to be deconstructed dispassionately, the way public high school students in the 1970s were expected to dissect pithed frogs marinated in formaldehyde?

The violations of trust are too numerous to count. Where there should have been institutional censure, Murray's professional peers bestowed upon him accolades and awards. He was never chastened by Harvard, nor anyone else.

In 1962, the year Murray retired, the American Psychological Association bestowed upon him the "Distinguished Scientific Contribution Award." The American Psychological Foundation honored him with its Gold Medal Award for Lifetime Achievement in the Application of Psychology. His experimental and clinical work became a de facto guide for modern clinical psychology. The dyad became clinical psychotherapy's operational model, which persists to this day. Despite Murray's claim that he was an impassioned and misunderstood visionary, his vision was nothing if not derivative. His therapeutic model followed Freud to a T, recreating the same unequal power relationship engendered by psychoanalysts: omniscient analyst, emotionally vulnerable patient who may as well be supine on a couch, even though psychotherapy as practiced in its modern iteration is generally conducted in chairs, with the patient and therapist facing each other.

All the same: The dyad is an autocracy. The patient must accept as part of the process the tenet that the therapist knows the patient better than the patient knows himself or herself.

The year after Murray completed his sadistic romp through Harvard's hapless male undergraduates, the Harvard Psilocybin Project commenced.

The Good Friday experiment, which occurred on Good Friday in April 1962 at Marsh Chapel at Boston University, could not have been more unlike Murray's experiment in philosophy, intention, or design. Other than both involving human beings, they were about as alike as chalk and cheese.

The architect and principal investigator, Walter N. Pahnke, was a thirty-one-year-old graduate student in religion and philosophy at the Harvard Graduate School of Arts and Sciences. The experiment, his PhD thesis project, titled "Drugs and Mysticism: An Analysis of the Relationship Between Psychedelic Drugs and the Mystical Consciousness," was the first double-blind study of psychoactive drugs and the mystical experience to be carried out in the United States.

It was not, however, the first clinical trial of psilocybin. Those first studies were conducted in France, four years prior.[20]

THE FIRST CLINICAL TRIALS WITH PSILOCYBIN, PARIS, 1958

In 1958, Dr. Jean Delay, president of the Faculty of Medicine at the main mental hospital in Paris, Centre Hospitalier Sainte-Anne, and the mycologist Roger Heim, director of the Muséum National d'Histoire Naturelle (MNHN), conducted a medical study on a group of thirteen "normal" subjects and thirty others who were characterized as "mentally ill." The subjects were given a total of fifty-two administrations of psilocybin. The very constrained purpose of the study was to provide "a descriptive presentation of the effects observed on the somatic and psychological level."[21] In other words, Heim and Delay were looking not for therapeutic effects but rather for any changes in physiological state (such as temperature, blood pressure, heart rate) and/ or changes in mental or emotional states (such as mood or the presence of hallucinations).

The first clinical trial of psilocybin as a therapeutic agent was conducted a year later, also in Paris, in 1959 by Dr. Anne-Marie Quétin for her PhD research.[22] The study was designed for the express purpose of treating psychiatric conditions with psilocybin. Earlier in the 1950s, Quétin's advisor, Delay, had overseen some of the most egregious examples of unethical misuse of LSD at Sainte-Anne on unsuspecting inmates, most of whom were women. His experiments amounted to torture: the hallucinogenic drug equivalent of Murray's experiment.

The psilocybin used in the early trials was formulated at Sandoz Laboratories in Basel, Switzerland, from mushrooms cultivated from spores of mycological samples collected by Heim and R. Gordon Wasson, an amateur mycologist and CIA asset, on research expeditions to Oaxaca, Mexico, in 1956.[23] The locale where identification of the active substance took place—Basel, rather than Paris, where the mushrooms containing the active compound originated—was the result of an unfortunate accident. A small amount of the active solution extracted from mushrooms cultivated at the museum was overturned onto the floor by a disgruntled museum chemist, Marcel Frèrejacques, who had been tasked by Heim with analyzing the active compound in the mushrooms. According to historian Vincent Verroust, Frèrejacques was not too keen on mycology, and the accident occurred.[24]

Rather than risk wasting further time on cultivation and extraction, Heim arranged for mushroom samples to be sent to Sandoz for analysis. There, Albert Hofmann, known as the father of LSD, and his colleagues identified, extracted, and synthesized the sacred mushrooms' active components: psilocybin and psilocin. Sandoz subsequently provided formulations of these substances in tablet and injectable liquid form to Delay in July 1958 for use at Sainte-Anne.[25]

Four years later, across the Atlantic, the first Anglo-Saxon experiment was conducted on the effects of psilocybin by doctoral candidate Dr. Walter Pahnke. His study was not about therapeutic medicine either, but rather about mystical consciousness and the spiritual experience.

The Good Friday Experiment

Walter Pahnke was born in 1931 in Harvey, Illinois, and attended Carleton College in Northfield, Minnesota.

By the time he carried out his PhD thesis project in 1962, Dr. Pahnke had earned an MD from Harvard in 1956, completed an internship in general medicine in Colorado, and received a second bachelor's degree, this one from Harvard Divinity School. Dr. Pahnke was not interested in the study of human behavior, nor was he interested in the kind of academic psychology on offer at Harvard. His focus on psychedelic drugs had to do with spirituality and religious experience. His goal was to explore their psychotherapeutic value, as well as their usefulness in the care of the dying.

Dr. William Richards, a clinical psychologist in the Department of Psychiatry at the Johns Hopkins University School of Medicine, met Dr. Pahnke in 1964 while both were training at the University of Göttingen in the therapeutic uses of LSD. They later became colleagues at Spring Grove State Hospital, in the Baltimore, Maryland, suburb of Catonsville. Richards described Dr. Pahnke as "an exceptionally brilliant man with impeccable integrity."

The Good Friday experiment was carried out under the supervision of Leary as part of the Harvard Psilocybin Project at the Harvard Center for Research in Personality. Leary had originated a previous study on psilocybin—the Concord Prison Experiment—as well as the better-known "Americans and Mushrooms in a Naturalistic Environment," for which the only recorded documentation is a single, unpublished, nine-page typescript.[26] The latter experiment involved Leary and his colleague, Richard Alpert (later known as Ram Dass), who was an assistant professor of clinical psychology, giving psilocybin to graduate students and volunteers in the community at large and asking them to document the experience.

The Concord Prison Experiment was an auspicious undertaking. Conducted between 1961 and 1963 in Concord State Prison, a maximum-security prison for young offenders, in Concord, Massachusetts, the study involved the administration of psilocybin to thirty-two prisoners in a group psychotherapy setting in an effort to reduce recidivism rates following their release. According to Leary's assessments, 88 percent of the subjects in the preliminary study reported that they learned something of value about themselves and 62 percent said that the experience of psilocybin changed their lives for the better. Some said psilocybin produced a "mystical" or "transcendent" experience similar to experiences of religious conversion.

Based upon this preliminary evidence, Leary speculated that the psilocybin experiences might be powerful catalysts of behavior change. In 1963, Leary reported recidivism rates to be reduced by 32 percent, slightly more than half of what was expected, 52 percent. A 1998 follow-up showed these figures to be misleading.[27] The key missing element, wrote follow-up author Rick Doblin, founder and executive director of the Multidisciplinary Association for Psychedelic Studies (MAPS), was the absence of "a comprehensive treatment plan that includes post-release, non-drug support programs." In other words, psilocybin experiences result in long-lasting emotional and behavioral changes only when the transcendent psilocybin experiences are integrated effectively into ordinary life through follow-up therapy.

Dr. Pahnke recruited the Good Friday experiment subjects, all students at the Andover Newton Theological Seminary, during a lecture on the Concord Prison Experiment. With the permission of Andover Newton, the students were offered the opportunity to have a personal experience with psilocybin after meeting with Dr. Pahnke.[28]

At the meeting, the volunteers were briefed on protocol and encouraged to ask questions. They were given a questionnaire to assess personal religious background, church affiliation, conversion experiences, mystical experience, and devotional life. Dr. Pahnke interviewed each volunteer for two hours prior to the experiment, questioning each about metabolic disease, drug and alcohol consumption, tobacco use, family history of mental illness, depression, whether they were in psychotherapy, and whether they suffered from symptoms of hysteria. Each subject was asked to interpret the meaning of the proverb "A rolling stone gathers no moss" in order to check on their fundamental abstract-reasoning power. Physical exams were performed. Suggestibility was tested by having the volunteers stand with their eyes closed, imagining that a strong wind was pushing them backward.

The volunteers were given a written summary of the anticipated program for the experiment. Dr. Pahnke then made suggestions for individual preparation: self-examination, meditation, private devotional life, or reading meaningful literature.

The subjects were divided into five groups of four and assigned two group leaders, all of whom were affiliated with the Harvard Psilocybin Project.

"The chief purpose of these leaders was to aid in creating a friendly and trust-filled set and setting which, it was hoped, would maximize the potential for positive experience, and to manage with confidence any disturbing reactions which might occur," wrote Dr. Pahnke.[29]

Half of the volunteers would receive an active dose, while the others would receive a dose of nicotinic acid (niacin); a leader was assigned to each subject receiving psilocybin. The groups met with their leaders for two hours prior to Good Friday "to develop group spirit and to prepare subjects for as positive and meaningful an experience as possible."[30]

On Good Friday 1962, the twenty divinity school students and ten group leaders, as well as two additional volunteers, religious scholar Huston Smith, who was teaching philosophy at the Massachusetts Institute of Technology at the time, and Walter Houston Clark, a professor of the psychology of religion at Andover Newton, gathered in a downstairs prayer room at Boston University's Marsh Chapel. Two smaller rooms furnished with sofas and chairs were made available. Candles were lit on the altar, which was set in front of three stained-glass windows. All but one of the lower chapel's three exits were locked. Shortly after 10:30 a.m., a helper who was not participating in the experiment handed out to each of the subjects an envelope containing either a capsule of 30 milligrams of psilocybin or a placebo. Each subject took the capsule with a cup of water.

For the next eighty minutes, the groups maintained silence. Subjects read, meditated, or prayed. The leaders were available to help anyone who experienced untoward effects such as nausea.

At 11:45 a.m., a bell was rung and the groups moved from the prayer room into the basement chapel. The minister, Howard Thurman, entered and welcomed the volunteers before heading upstairs to start the Good Friday service, which commenced with an organ prelude. Loudspeakers broadcast the Mass from the main sanctuary to the chapel and rooms below.

Dr. Pahnke remained outside the chapel, emergency medical kit at the ready.

At 2:30 p.m., when the service ended, the groups remained in the chapel. Group leaders escorted subjects one at a time into one of the smaller meeting rooms, where each participant was asked to describe his experience on tape, while the other leader stayed behind with the rest of the group.

Participants scored their experience by category, including transcendence of time and space, dissolution of the self in relationship to the world, transiency, paradoxicality, and persisting positive changes toward self and life.

One of the participants, identified as RM, described his experience of ego dissolution. "I saw the cosmos. It was all molten plastic. I knew that I must be somewhere there. Where was my self? What am I? Where am I in the real (plastic) world? Then I was afraid no more. My self is no one place but in many places. It floats, I float. Body is not real. Only the adventurous self is real. The adventurous self floats into all Being, the orange plastic cosmos. It leaves the old ego behind. The old ego is behind but it glows like a faraway harbor light. I can always return."[31]

All but one of those who took part in the experiment and received clinical doses described the experience as one of the most transformative, important of their lives.

Participant TB, on being interviewed for the follow-up study, said, "I can think of no experiences [like the Good Friday experience] quite of that magnitude."

Participant FK experienced what could be characterized as a "bad trip," a response, so it appeared to Huston Smith, to the contents of Reverend Thurman's sermon. A few minutes into the service, FK got up and went to the altar. Then, instead of returning and sitting down, he marched to the rear entrance of the chapel and exited. In an interview, Smith, who realized something was amiss when FK didn't return to his pew, recalled the incident in detail.

"He had made a right turn and was striding down the hall, but we had been told that the entire basement had been sealed off for the experiment, so I was not overly concerned. But when he reached the door at the end of the corridor and jammed down its latch bar, it swung open. Something had misfired in the instructions to the janitor, and my charge, zonked out of his skull, was at large on Commonwealth Avenue. I ran after him, but my urgings to return to the chapel fell on deaf ears, and he shook off my grip on his elbow as if it were cobwebs."[32]

Ultimately, FK was subdued by Smith, Dr. Pahnke, and a team leader and taken back to the chapel, where Dr. Pahnke injected him with a dose of chlorpromazine, an antipsychotic that is used as a sedative and a tranquilizer. At first, he could not remember anything about the incident. But, twenty-four hours later, he recalled what had taken place. He said he had left the chapel because God had chosen him to announce to the world the dawning of a millennium of peace and goodwill, which he needed to deliver to the world at large.

When asked to participate in Doblin's long-term follow-up, FK declined. His memory of the experience was almost entirely negative, so much so that he threatened to sue Doblin should his name be used in any published material.

Another subject, SJ, on being interviewed for the follow-up study, said, "Something extraordinary had taken place which had never taken place before. All of a sudden, I felt sort of drawn out into infinity, and all of a sudden, I had lost touch with my mind. I felt that I was caught up in the vastness of Creation . . . huge as the mystics say. . . . I did experience that kind of classic kind of blending . . . Sometimes you would look up and see the light on the altar and it would just be a blinding sort of light and radiation. . . . That main thing about it was a sense of timelessness."[33]

Following the completion of his experiment and the submission of his thesis, Dr. Pahnke departed for the Georg-August University in Göttingen, Germany, to train with Hanscarl Leuner in LSD-assisted psychotherapy. On his return to the United States, Dr. Pahnke worked at the Massachusetts Mental Health Center in Boston, and then went on to psychedelic therapy work at Spring Grove State Hospital. He eventually became director of clinical sciences at the Maryland Psychiatric Research Center and assistant professor of psychiatry at the Johns Hopkins University School of Medicine.

Despite its success, the Good Friday experiment did not augur well for Leary or Alpert. The Harvard Psilocybin Project's ultimate failure had nothing to do with either the scientific or anecdotal evidence Dr. Pahnke's research had yielded. Far from it. The problem lay squarely with the leadership style of the project's faculty overseers.

Leary and Alpert had become increasingly lax about the screening of participants they recruited for the "Americans and Mushrooms in a Naturalistic Environment" project. In an editorial in *The Harvard Crimson*, Harvard University officials asserted, "Far from exercising the caution that characterizes the public statements of most scientists, Leary and Alpert, in their papers and speeches, have been given to making the kind of pronouncements about their work that one associates with quacks."[34]

In April 1962, the Massachusetts Food and Drugs Division began an investigation of the research. Their findings concluded that Leary and Alpert had failed to have physicians present when drugs were administered, which was a legal requirement. A faculty committee was appointed to "advise and oversee" future studies of psilocybin. Neither of these fixes produced the intended consequences. There was little if any oversight. Things got worse.

"The shoddiness of their work as scientists is the result less of incompetence than of a conscious rejection of scientific ways of looking at things," zinged the *Crimson* in an editorial. "Leary and Alpert fancy themselves prophets of a psychic revolution designed to free Western man from the limitations of consciousness as we know it. They are contemptuous of all organized systems of action—of what they call the 'roles' and 'games' of society. They have not been professors at Harvard—they have been playing 'the professor game,' and their cynicism has led them to disregard University regulations and standards of good faith. They have violated the one condition Harvard placed upon their work; that they not use undergraduates as subjects for drug experiments."[35]

By the time Alpert was dismissed from his academic appointment for giving "consciousness-expanding drugs" to undergraduates, Leary had already abandoned ship. He was relieved of his duties when he left Cambridge without notice and failed to show up to teach. His contract was terminated on April 30, 1963.

In 1971, in response to the bad press out of Harvard and the increasingly widespread street use of psychoactive drugs, psilocybin, heroin, LSD, and marijuana were all summarily placed on Schedule 1 of the Controlled Substances Act, which identifies these substances as having high potential for abuse and no accepted medical use in the United States. Practitioners like Richards, who had watched the clinical benefits of psilocybin and LSD unfold on a daily basis in his work at Spring Grove State Hospital and the Maryland Psychiatric Research Center, now found their work being summarily dismissed. By this time, much of the work being done with psilocybin and LSD revolved around treatment and alleviation of anxiety and depression in the terminally ill.

Dr. Pahnke didn't live long enough to witness the destiny of his life's work. Unlike Richards—and the many patients who might have benefited from treatment with psychoactive drugs—he did not have to witness the consequences of its banishment.

On a clear July day in 1971, at the age of forty, Dr. Pahnke, trying out scuba diving for the first time, dove underwater just yards from his family holiday home at the seaside near Bath, Maine. He never emerged, and his remains were never found, despite an extended search.

Of his life, Richards said, "He had a great sense of humor and he was also impulsive. If he'd have waited two minutes for Eva [his wife] to come out of the house and join him, which she was going to do, he'd be alive. If Wally turned out to be alive after all these years, as some maintain he is, living someplace in South America, the first thing I'd do if I saw him would be to give him a huge hug. Then I'd give him an equally swift kick in the backside."

More to the point than his impulsivity, however, was the loss to the world of Dr. Pahnke's visionary work, his profound sense of humanity, and his calling to restore a sense of life's meaning to those who are terminally ill.

In 1968, while working at the Maryland Psychiatric Research Center, Dr. Pahnke was invited to deliver the Ingersoll Lecture on human immortality, an annual Harvard University event in which a distinguished researcher or philosopher in the field is invited to speak. In an ensuing article discussing giving LSD to terminally ill cancer patients, Dr. Pahnke wrote:

> The most dramatic effects came in the wake of a psychedelic mystical experience. There was a decrease in fear, anxiety, worry, and depression. Sometimes the need for pain medications was lessened, but mainly because the patient was able to tolerate what pain he had more easily. There was an increase in serenity, peace, and calmness. Most striking was a decrease in the fear of death. It seems as if the mystical experience, by opening the patient to usually untapped ranges of human consciousness, can provide a sense of security that transcends even death. Once the patient is able to release all the psychic energy which he has tied to the fear of death and worry about the future, he seems able to live more meaningfully in the present. He can turn his attention to the things which have the most significance in the here and now. This change of attitude has an effect on all the people around him. The depth and intensity of interpersonal closeness can be increased so that honesty and courage emerge in a joint confrontation and acceptance of the total situation.[36]

The response of the Nixon administration was predictably untethered. The last thing they were interested in was humanistic medicine. In 1971, the Justice Department decreed psilocybin and LSD along with a number of other drugs to have no accepted medical use.

What can we make of the real-world outcomes of these experiments? Harvard and the psychological establishment cheerfully lauding Murray's morally reprehensible research, while summarily condemning the work of Leary, Alpert, and ultimately Dr. Pahnke? What conclusions can we draw?

If we take personalities out of the picture, which given the power of each of them is hard to do, we are left with institutions and post-Enlightenment power structures. A Moby Dick analogy may be useful here.

The white whale, Moby Dick, whom the captain of the whaler *Pequod*, Captain Ahab, is desperate to vanquish, symbolizes the powerful and unstoppable forces of nature. The captain's sole mission in life is to destroy the great white whale who had relieved him of his leg. He is willing to rout and kill anything and anyone in order to do it. He's the personification of post-Enlightenment industrial society. He is the Enlightenment conquistador, and it is nature itself he desperately needs to conquer.

Murray was blind to Moby Dick's more obvious parallels. Although he stalwartly thought of himself as an intellectual outsider, Murray existed within the institutional structures of modern psychology, modern medicine, modern society, and modern academia. He was an unalloyed piece of the architecture, and he was a miserable failure at observing, much less comprehending, the bricks and mortar he himself inhabited.

Leary and Alpert—and, by extension, Dr. Pahnke—embodied the forces of nature. To the institutions of Harvard, the State of Massachusetts, and, ultimately, the US government, they were the adversary. They were the whale. Their work represented the mystical, unstoppable forces of nature. They did not want to master and destroy the human psyche; they wanted to celebrate and integrate it and, in so doing, lift mankind itself into a nobler existence. They represented everything the Enlightenment had tried to annihilate. They valued learning unrelated to the academy and culture as it existed at 1960s Harvard.

Murray and his ilk lived according to a credo that demanded autocratic relationships; concentrated top-down power hierarchies; affirmed received knowledge to the exclusion of anything else; annihilated imagination; and relied wholly on scientific positivism to explain the natural world. As far as compassion for the human experience was concerned, he could not have even faked it.

As I write this, years after the fact, it's plain to me that the psychology Murray engendered, practiced, cultivated, and propagated through his enormous influence in the field is at least partly to blame for laying the social and psychosocial groundwork for the worldwide neofascist upsurge we're now undergoing. His philosophy was less about personhood, where sentient beings with a vast color palette of emotions and feelings evolve through a lifetime of relationships and life experiences, than it was one of personality fetishism. From Murray's vantage point, other humans were lesser beings than he. He turned them dispassionately into commodities for the sake of his own career, useful only insofar as they could aid and abet him in serving the goals of his own massive ego. His was the psychology of narcissism.

My parents, as part of the same machine that produced Murray and the generations of psychologists and psychiatrists who followed, were perfect expressions of his approach to the human experience. My parents' denial of the alcoholism, violence, and generational pedophilia within the family served the same dangerous personal and professional ethos. Both my parents and Murray caused the loss of life of those around them. They suffered no consequences.

When I saw her shortly before she died, my sister Andrea told me she thought she'd never have gotten married if she hadn't gone into therapy to get herself untangled from our parents' influence. She identified my father as the clear bad guy. I didn't argue, although I told her that she and I had entirely different experiences of our parents, which is the pattern in dysfunctional families where the interpersonal dynamics are governed by violent abuse and alcoholism.

Then she said, "I always thought you thought one of us had been molested as a child."

I did not push the point with her. I realized at that moment her therapist could never have dreamed of addressing the possibility that her problems stemmed from childhood sexual abuse. Even at that late stage, she was still extremely overweight—not, she told me, as overweight as she had been a few years prior when she was "really fat."

Later, after the meeting—our last—I cried for hours. *If she'd had a therapist who had not been part of the same cabal as every other psychotherapist trained in the neo-Freudian model, she would not be dying.* Her obesity would have been addressed; she would have received real medical care; and the tumor would have been identified long before it was terminal.

In contrast to Murray and his brethren, Leary, Alpert, and Dr. Pahnke reveled in relationships based on equality and mutual respect. They believed in communal rather than hierarchical social structures. They viewed knowledge gained in ways not defined by or within institutional structures as authentic, true, and far more valuable than pedantry. They had an abundance of imagination and they believed in a transcendent spirituality. They had profound compassion and respect for human experience.

No wonder Harvard—and the institutions of government, medicine, psychiatry, and business—reviled everything the psychedelic drug experimenters stood for. Personified by Nixon and later on by Reagan and subsequent leaders around the world, American institutions adopted this idiotic and paradoxical stance without a trace of irony. Neofascism was emerging as the predominant social and political ideology.

A lifetime later, with the recent reentry of psychedelics on the therapeutic scene, when everything should have changed, when the age of human progress should have been well underway, the situation has gotten only worse. Not just worse, dire. Now psychedelics are ballyhooed by zealots and marketed by tech bros and fake journalists who are no more than shills for the pharmaceutical industry. The worst elements among these are the American capitalists, whose presence as influencers in this scene does not bode well. The *nous* of the psychedelic experience—psychedelics consumed within a cultural and spiritual context—is lost. Reinventing psychedelics as pharmaceutical drugs mangles the transcendent meaning of the experiences they engender and ejects the once-sacred catalytic substances—such as psilocybin—into the voracious, spiritually and intellectually bankrupt maw of the post-Enlightenment industrial elite. Set and setting, ritual context, a compassionate group of fellow villagers within a community wherein the experiences are processed and incorporated into everyday life will be eliminated in favor of profit making on the part of the pharmaceutical guilds, which have already set in motion a vision of psilocybin as the new "mother's little helper," the nickname for the drug diazepam (Valium), the anxiolytic and sedative. And there's the Silicon Valley version, psychedelics as daily performance enhancers for a generation of emotionally challenged young men, small doses of psilocybin that can be used to whisk them to the head of the pack in the soul-murdering institution of American industry.

CHAPTER 4

NEUROTRANSMITTERS AND THE FALLACY OF THE MAGIC PILL

My first experience with prescribed psychotropic drugs occurred when I was in graduate school at Brown University. I was in an MA program in the English Department, a creative writing program. I was a top student. I had a decent and well-intended boyfriend. A few weeks into my second semester, I received a call from the Dean of Students' office. I owed that semester's tuition. I would not be able to enroll the following year if I didn't find a way to pay it. The news was a gut punch. I went to see the dean. It emerged that my father had arranged to have the need-based portion of my financing package rescinded my second semester by entering me as a dependent on his taxes.

I'd been financially independent for over a year by then. The rest of my tuition and small stipend were paid by dint of a merit-based scholarship. According to Brown's calculations, I no longer qualified for the need-based portion. I broke down in the office. The dean suggested I call my parents; perhaps it was a mistake. The call, which I did not want to make, was useless. You see, he needed the money. He had to pay Andrea's tuition. By then, Andrea was a freshman at Vassar College. He offered to send me $400 per month instead. To cover rent. I already knew how this form of abuse would play out. It was a game in which I was to pretend he was not abusing me, a game played on me, at my expense, so he could engage in a charade of caring father while robbing me of something he knew I desperately needed. A dash of signature Leiderman sadism: He finessed the project by pitting my needs against those of my sister.

I managed to obtain an emergency loan for $100 from the graduate school—enough to buy groceries, but not nearly enough to cover the tuition.

I applied for a student loan.

That year, I began publishing stories. A year later, I wrote the short story that would win me a National Magazine Award.

After a month, an envelope with a check for $400 arrived in the mail. I cashed it. It was stopped, leaving me with an overdraft on my account. The following month, no check. Then, six weeks later, an envelope with a pink index card and the words "Andrea's tuition" scrawled on it. The following month, another pink index card with the letters "I O U" scrawled on it.

I was afraid to tell my boyfriend, R, about my scholarship. I was afraid even to see him. I didn't want him to feel as though he had to pay for groceries.

Unlike my parents, R's mother wasn't educated. She had lived her entire life in a small southern New Hampshire rust-belt town. She'd raised six kids on her own after R's dad died of throat cancer when R was eleven. They were on public assistance until she got a job as a dispatcher for the local police department. She remained there for the rest of her working life. I spent Christmas with him. I was awestruck by R's ma, her profound kindness and generosity. Even though she'd never met me, she had bought me gifts so I, too, would have "something under the tree."

I was mortified at Christmas dinner when the wine I'd brought as a gift at first couldn't be opened for want of a corkscrew. They didn't have one in the house because the wine they were accustomed to came with screw tops. Eventually, one was borrowed from a neighbor.

R was the first in his family to obtain an advanced degree. He was on a Federal Pell Grant. At Brown, R lived in a group house with several roommates not far from where I lived. R's mother, who knew he was living on a shoestring, would send him checks now and then, $20 here, $50 there—not only for him but also so that we could go out to dinner or go away for the weekend. I was too ashamed at the time to tell him about what had become of my scholarship. Not understanding the dynamics of my family, he viewed my parents' status as aspirational. I, on the other hand, wanted to flee from that background and way of life as fast as my feet would carry me. I had not yet figured out how to do it. I felt nothing but shame.

The theme of shame recurs for abused women: We take on what was done as though it were something we did to ourselves. The abusers are the victims. The shame becomes ours.

One day, my father decided to show up in Providence. He announced his intentions as an edict with little notice, declaring he would take me and my friends out for drinks at the Biltmore Hotel, a formerly upscale hotel that had become a little seedy. I remember R at my apartment asking whether I wanted him to join. The tension my father brought with him was almost unbearable. I told R I didn't want to subject him to it, unless he thought he could stand it. R, for his part, was offended. He felt I was judging him, as though I thought he was not good enough. The opposite was true, and I'm ashamed to this day I was so incompetent at articulating it. I wanted to protect him from what I knew would transpire. I wanted to protect him from my father.

I don't recall much of what happened, other than my father flirting with my embarrassed roommates, who joined us, and R trying very hard to find a topic with which to engage my father that wasn't abusively dismissed. Ever game, R finally tried politics. John Anderson was running for president. He got my father to respond to that.

Years later, R recalled the incident, saying, "I didn't really give a flying fuck how he was treating me; what really made me mad was the way he treated you. This beautiful, accomplished, gracious daughter, and he was just beating the shit out of you in front of your friends. I'd never seen anything like it."

I could not tell him how things really were in my family of origin, and he stopped trying to reconcile what he'd seen with what he wanted and what he was hoping to have with me. My relationship filled me with anxiety.

Weeks went by and I could not sleep. I went to the student health center, where the consulting psychologist prescribed a round of clorazepate dipotassium (Tranxene), an antianxiety agent. The sleeplessness was only the beginning of what became an emotional avalanche. I wasn't living; I was faking it. I wasn't a person; I was a projection of a person I desperately wanted to be. My very being was as fragile as a cracked Fabergé egg. One slight wrong move, one tiny thing out of place, I would break open and shatter into a million pieces. I held myself together, more or less, through graduation. After that I completely fell apart.

It was at Brown, where I was liked and admired by people well outside of my parents' universe, that the impact of my childhood of nighttime beatings, of abuse, of gaslighting, of terror at the hands of my parents, began to bubble to the surface.

But the real nadir of my chronic post-traumatic stress disorder (CPTSD), when events forced me to confront how estranged I'd become from my physical body, to say nothing of my emotions, and how far my very soul had fled, didn't occur when I was in grad school. The precipitating events, and the ensuing smashing open of the Pandora's box where my childhood was stashed, occurred a few years earlier, before I went to Brown, while I was in college and the year after I graduated.

Back in 1980, nothing was known about CPTSD. It didn't even have a name until 1992, when Dr. Judith Herman identified it as distinct and separate from PTSD. The epigenetic, physiological, disease-causing component was identified much later.

CPTSD is not just psychological, a problem of mood or affect played out in emotional or behavioral ways and easily treated with an antidepressant or anxiolytic medication, perhaps a bit of cognitive behavioral therapy (CBT) thrown in for good measure. Childhood violence resulting in CPTSD is a whole-body, whole-brain physiological injury to the organism, from nervous system to skeleton, from which one never fully recovers.

I am someone who manages life with a chronic, life-threatening illness the way those with type 1 diabetes manage, knowing they're only a few insulin doses away from death. I've developed strategies and habits for organizing my life so that I don't become emotionally dysregulated—fearful, frightened, anxious—or find myself resorting to some kind of compulsive activity to control my mood or my environment. Or, as has often happened, suddenly dissociating in a situation where my life or well-being may be endangered. It is imperative I remain in the present moment and do not dissociate. I keep a regular schedule. I try to get lots of exercise, mostly now through yoga. I meditate. I do not allow any alcohol or drug abusers into my life. I look through narcissists as if they don't exist. I avoid gluttons at all costs. I work at not becoming thoroughly isolated.

With each repeated act of violence when I was a young child, with every threat of sphincter-loosening, vomit-inducing terror, a bit more of the integrated whole was torn away, layer by irreplaceable layer. The repeated assaults on my senses corroded my health the way acid dripped steadily onto a padlock eventually cuts through it.

Whereas trauma confined to individual incidents allows the body and the mind time and space to rebound, ongoing, unhalting physical and psychological violence does not. There is no room to heal. There is no time-out space. The changes are etched into the very essence of the body and the mind.

The impairment to an organism's ability to reregulate physiological and psychological processes brought on by constant and repetitive violence has been documented extensively in the literature. Childhood trauma is associated with disruptions in activity of the hypothalamic–pituitary–adrenal (HPA) axis, which is the main stress-response system. The adrenal cortex and the so-called stress hormone cortisol are part of this axis. When the axis malfunctions, the cascade of physiological events that ensues causes an endless array of health sequelae later in life.

The HPA axis is the neuroendocrine link between stress or trauma as we experience it and the somatic response to stress. The bath of cortisol released during the experience of ongoing or repeated traumatic events in childhood, such as physical or sexual abuse, causes changes to the resiliency of the HPA axis through an epigenetic change called DNA methylation. DNA methylation is a disease-promoting genetic modification affecting gene expression. DNA methylation in the HPA system leads to a sequence of biochemical events, which cause disruption in neuroendocrine, behavioral, autonomic, and metabolic functions in adulthood. This disruption is the direct epigenetic link between childhood trauma and mental, emotional, and physical illness.[1]

Cancer is among the many diseases associated with DNA methylation.[2] Cortisol-induced HPA axis malfunctions disrupt the biological mechanism that prevents DNA methylation. Once this mechanism is dismantled, there is nothing to interfere with DNA methylation in the body, and there is nothing to prevent normal biological processes such as cell replication, or immune response, from going off the rails.

Even though I did not know anything at the time about psychotropic drugs and how they work on the brain or how the violence in my childhood was really affecting me, I knew Tranxene wasn't going to fix it. But who wanted to find out what the real underlying problems were? I'd been trained in the art of the masquerade. Twenty-three years of gaslighting had gotten me there.

I'd been led to believe the reason I could not sleep and was hyper-reactive to every kind of emotional stress was my problem to bear. Endopsychic, reflective of a flawed self.

When I think about psychotropics and CPTSD, what comes to mind is the Mad Tea-Party from *Alice's Adventures in Wonderland*, by itself one of the wackiest scenes in modern (nonclassical) literature. The scene takes place during a tea party, at which Alice, the March Hare, the Hatter, and the Dormouse are seated at a table set for tea. The Hatter's watch is broken. The Hatter and the March Hare are having an altercation over the March Hare's attempt to repair it by buttering the caliber. When the Hatter fumes he'd told the Hare not to butter the watch, the March Hare protests meekly, "It was the *best* butter." The best butter should be able to fix anything, shouldn't it?

The best pharmaceutical drugs were not going to repair the workings of a mind and body that had been in a state of prolonged abuse any more than the best butter was going to repair the Hatter's watch. The butter does what butter does best, in its universe of tea and crumpets. It has nothing to do with the watch. Pharmaceutical drugs for the mind are *sui generis*, in a universe of their own, created primarily to butter the bank accounts of those who invest in them. They have nothing to do with the soul, the spirit, or the well-being of the humans who are instructed to ingest them.

The Tranxene nostrum helped me sleep for a few weeks, but it wasn't even a Band-Aid, any more than a tourniquet tied on the severed stump of an arm has anything to do with rejoining what remains of the bloody appendage dangling by a thread of skin below the elbow. My second year at Brown, I knew the Fabergé egg was well and truly falling apart. By the time I finished my MA, I was dissociating. I couldn't tell whether what I felt was happening now, in the present, or was something that had happened twenty years before. I didn't sleep for nights on end. Conflict terrified me. I didn't understand normal anger, normal fear, or, above all, real affection.

I couldn't commit. I broke up with R because I knew I'd never be able to hold it together in a relationship, although the friendship continued for decades. I was afraid if I got married and had a baby, I'd abuse my children. He wanted to move in together; he wanted to start a family. There had been a brief moment when I thought I might be pregnant. Rather than outrage, he expressed happiness. But for me, anything that looked, talked, walked, or smelled like family terrified me. I couldn't tell him what had happened in my childhood until years later, when we were in our thirties. Some part of me feared that anyone who knew what had happened would see me as fundamentally and irretrievably broken and flawed. I figured I was condemned to a life of separateness. It was probably best just to bow out of relationships until I could find a way to glue myself together. Managing to stay in the present at all during my time at Brown was something of a miracle, an act of will.

The very idea that a pill, or a series of pills, or a lifetime of pills could even touch the fallout from my formative years was risible. By then, though, the pharmaceutical industry was already barreling along, and the pill version of "mental health" was well on its way to taking over the practice of psychiatry.

The *DSM*, Pill Pushing, and the Killing of Normal

The bible of psychoactive pill pushers everywhere, the *Diagnostic and Statistical Manual of Mental Disorders*, now in its fifth edition, is consistently on best-seller lists. As of this writing, it is the number one best seller on Amazon in the psychiatry category and that is in spite of the price: The paperback edition of the *DSM-5* costs a whopping $99. The book's best-seller status should come as no surprise: The pharmaceutical industry buys the *DSM* in bulk and then provides drug salesmen free copies to give as gifts to clinicians when they make sales calls to doctors' offices. The popularity of the book is calculated, willful, and artificial. But by pharmaceutical lights, handing out this tome like a party favor is just good business. It drives up diagnosis rates and promotes the writing of prescriptions for medications.[3]

By the time the *DSM-5* came into being, the belief that a daily pill could do what a lifetime on the couch could not, had already taken hold in American psychiatry. Psychoanalysis was moribund. Drive theory was not exactly a viable contestant in this peculiar version of pro wrestling, wherein the emerging and commercially unstoppable field of psychopharmacology lurked Hulk Hogan–like as the enemy combatant in the opposite corner.[4] And psychedelics had entirely disappeared from the medical scene, banished to the netherworld of drug scheduling, contraband substances, and a small but stalwart psychedelic underground who continued to practice furtively, out of sight from mainstream medicine.

The *DSM-5* and its predecessors were the outgrowth of an attempt on the part of the US government to gather information about mental health in the United States, producing, in the 1840 census, a description of the frequency of "idiocy/insanity" in the population, according to the website of the American Psychiatric Association (APA).

By the 1880 census, seven categories of mental health were distinguished: mania, melancholia, monomania, paresis, dementia, dipsomania, and epilepsy. From then on, the effort to classify mental disorders—and presumably to treat them—took on a life of its own.

One of the most telling details about the progression of mental health—or maybe about the degradation of mental health in service of the medical and pharmaceutical industries—was a single word change that occurred between the creation of the first *DSM* (previously cataloged under the mental-disorders section of the International Classification of Diseases or ICD) and the second, *DSM-II*: the purging of the word *reaction*. During this time, British psychiatrist Erwin Stengel was enlisted by the World Health Organization (WHO) to review diagnostic criteria in the

ICD and address the need for "explicit definitions of disorders as a means of promoting reliable clinical diagnoses."[5] Although his report motivated many advances, during the next round of revisions, the editors "did not follow Stengel's recommendations to any great degree. *DSM-II* was similar to *DSM* but eliminated the term 'reaction.'"[6]

What does elimination of the word *reaction* signify? Why is that word important? It is important for this reason: From 1968 on, mental disorders were no longer considered to be reactive, according to the diagnostic criteria. Sadness, fear, regret, apprehension, and cognitive dysfunction were no longer considered to be normal reactions to major events in a person's life to which a person has an emotionally healthy response. In a time and place where lived experience was respected, responses to a loved one's death that included crying, renting of clothing, and tearing of hair, followed by malaise and inability to eat or sleep, would have been considered signs that the brain was firing on all cylinders. The *DSM-II* changed all that. This singular, linguistic sleight of hand did for the pharmaceutical industry expansion mission what medical psychiatry has done since the 1890s: blame the patient for the circumstances of their own trauma, anxiety, mania, depression, or—as in the case of Freud's patient Emma Eckstein—near-fatal iatrogenic nosebleed.[7] The adjective *iatrogenic* is very useful. Its origin is ancient Greek: ιατρός = *doctor* + γένεσις = *genesis*, or: "the doctor made the disease."

Removal of the concept of reactivity from mental health diagnostic criteria unlatched any notion of environmental factors or public health or personal trauma, such as childhood abuse, from clinical assessments and stuck it squarely inside the head of the sufferer. Your unhappiness or emotional distress is a symptom of your own pathology. Since then, unsurprisingly, the medical, psychiatric, and pharmaceutical guilds, which produced successive editions of the *DSM*, have done nothing to improve mental health outcomes. Instead, outcomes have become astronomically worse.

The *DSM* is anything but a scientifically sound diagnostic standard. At best, it is a reflection of the priorities of its creators. The most recent version of the *DSM*, a 947-page tome, titled *DSM-5*, contains descriptions of approximately 370 diagnosable psychiatric disorders. It provides, according to the APA website, "the field with a summary of the state of the science relevant to psychiatric diagnosis and letting it know where gaps existed in the current research."[8] However, the description masks a more avaricious reality about the motivations of the book's creators. According to an article in *New Scientist*, most of the psychiatrists (57 percent) who wrote the *DSM-5* had ties to the pharmaceutical industry.[9] The difference between this volume and previous volumes was that, for the first time in its history, contributors were required to produce disclosure statements. Authors had to declare their financial ties to industry. They could receive up to $10,000 from drug companies in a year; their stockholding in pharmaceutical companies could amount to no more than $50,000. The worst part, however, was not the amount they had at stake but rather their inordinate influence on what constituted a legitimate diagnosis. Those with ties to industry were describing illnesses and altering diagnostic categories for disorders that were considered especially controversial. The mood disorders group, for instance, proposed the inclusion of bereavement in the definition of major depression—as though grief were an illness rather than a normal response to a terrible, demoralizing event: the death of a loved one. In 2022—just in time for much of the world's timid emergence from COVID-19—"prolonged grief disorder" was declared an illness and added to the *DSM*.

The psychotic disorders group was considering adding "attenuated psychosis syndrome," described in the *New Scientist* article as "a controversial diagnosis for identifying young people *at risk of developing schizophrenia*" (emphasis mine).[10] Circling like vultures around a new, lucrative population to exploit pharmaceutically, they were, by including this new category, recruiting clinicians to profile young people who *had not developed symptoms of any mental illness* in service of diagnosing them with nonexistent illness, because an *illness may follow.*

The "pre-diagnosis" gives them license to pre-prescribe an antipsychotic medication that will, if current patterns continue to play out, have dire effects on these young people's lives years down the road. This bizarre reasoning reminds me of the 2002 film *The Minority Report*, in which a police crime-fighting unit apprehends criminals before they commit crimes using the prescient powers of three psychics.[11]

By designating what constitutes mental illness and selecting whom to label with a diagnosis, *DSM* psychiatrists—through public appearances and lectures—also influence who prescribes what. They're paid by pharmaceutical companies to flog products to prescribing doctors and medical institutions. A full 15 percent of work group members were found to be members of speakers bureaus.

Why is it, then, with all the pharmaceutical ammunition being turned out to cure us of our woes, do we find numbers like the following? The United States has the highest suicide rate of any wealthy nation. Suicides account for 14 deaths per 100,000 people. This is double the suicide rate of the United Kingdom. The US suicide rate climbed by over 33 percent from 1999 to 2018 while, globally, the suicide rate has dropped by 38 percent since the mid-1990s.

Meanwhile, according to the US Centers for Disease Control and Prevention (CDC), between 2015 and 2018, 13.2 percent of Americans aged eighteen and over reported having taken antidepressant medication in the prior thirty days. That is around 44.2 million people.

Antidepressant use was higher among women than men in every age group. Use increased with age, in both men and women. Almost one-quarter of women aged sixty and over (24.3 percent) took antidepressants.

In the UK, 7.3 million people, or 17 percent of the population, are prescribed antidepressants, according to the Prescribed

Medicines Review Summary, 2020. The economic and social cost of mental ill health in England has grown in the last decade to almost £119 billion ($149.3 billion) a year. In 2009, the figure was £105 billion ($131.8 billion).

These figures are both daunting and tragic. Over the course of the thirty-plus years—especially since the introduction of SSRIs—the medicalization of normal human emotional states has led to an epidemic of diagnoses and prescription writing. Far from becoming the mental health equivalent of penicillin or the polio vaccine—medical drugs that actually cure real disease—SSRIs created chronic recurrent illnesses out of problems that are most often transient in nature.

During this period, a huge amount of data has accumulated about the outcomes for patients taking these drugs over the long term. In country after country, study after study, evidence shows long-term use of psychiatric medication causes depression, mood disruption, and medical effects (such as akathisia, a movement disorder) that can be more problematic than the original diagnosis. Used for more than a few months, the drugs create more disease than they treat. Although patients may initially experience minor improvements, long-term use results in a steady, inexorable downward spiral in mental and emotional states.

Dr. James Davies, author of *Sedated: How Modern Capitalism Created Our Mental Health Crisis*, has explored this trend in detail, correlating it with a number of destructive societal trends, such as increased borrowing and unsecured debt. In the UK, for example, holding unsecured debt in the immediate aftermath of the Second World War was considered almost a moral failing.[12] But the rate of unsecured borrowing per household in Britain rose from about £2,600 in 1987 to £16,000 in 2019. As a percentage of household income, 10 percent of households were in some debt in 1987; by 2019 over 30 percent carried debt of close to £16,000.[13]

Davies puts it succinctly: "While each industry offers its own profitable elixir for emotional success, they all share and promote the same consumerist philosophy of suffering: your central problem is not that you've been mis-taught how to understand and engage with your difficulties . . . but the fact that you experience suffering at all—something that targeted consumption can address."[14]

In both the United States and Great Britain, people consume far more than they need yet are more dissatisfied than ever in their day-to-day lives. Davies makes the point that the correspondence between these two curves is no coincidence: There is an undeniable relationship between the neoliberal social and economic policies unleashed in both Great Britain and the United States during the Thatcher and Reagan eras of the 1980s and the catastrophic uptick in prescribing of psychiatric medication. In both countries, social and economic supports for people experiencing mental health problems were summarily defunded. The cost of mental health care was considered an unnecessary expense. Long-term care facilities providing supportive environments were closed and support structures for ordinary people were eroded. In Britain, Thatcher's signature move was to allow people to purchase their council houses—government-subsidized housing—at reduced rates, which decimated the stock of public housing available for people who still needed it.

Now on the open market, former council housing can be resold at a profit. Those who need subsidized housing can wait upward of five years for units to become available. Even poorer, they are less able than ever to get their social, health, and economic needs met. Electric service rates have risen to the point where many people are not able to heat their homes during the winter. To any sane person, this situation is deeply demoralizing. People who find themselves in it become desperate and accept the chemical cures they are given *because they are desperate*. Prescribing doctors are only too happy to dispense them.

SEROTONIN AND THE CHEMICAL-IMBALANCE THEORY OF DEPRESSION

The most-prescribed drugs for depression in the United States and in the UK by far are SSRIs, drugs used to prevent the reuptake of excess synaptic serotonin in the brain. Serotonin—5-hydroxytryptamine or 5-HT—is a neurotransmitter found in all regions of the body, especially in the gut and in blood, as well as in the brain, where it is produced in neurons originating in the raphe nuclei, located in the midline of the brain stem. Higher serotonin concentrations are found in the brain stem than in the cortex. SSRIs work by causing serotonin to accumulate in the synapses between neurons. These medications have been celebrated as major miracles in denting the fog of depression for millions of people around the globe, yet, as evidence has shown over the last thirty years, their prolonged use damages the proper functioning of the brain and, along with it, the lives of most of the patients who have consumed them long term. The only real beneficiaries of this epidemic of overprescribing and use have been the pharmaceutical companies and psychiatrists with lucrative ties to industry.

Originally identified in 1935 by Vittorio Erspamer, an Italian pharmacologist and chemist, serotonin is a vasoconstrictive monoamine found in the gastrointestinal tracts of vertebrates and in organs of several invertebrates. Vasoconstrictors are chemical compounds that cause the small muscles around blood vessels to tighten, reducing blood flow. In 1949, the chemical composition of a vasoconstrictive indolealkylamine, 5-hydroxytryptamine (5-HT or serotonin) was identified in red blood cells, the same vasoconstrictor Erspamer had identified years before.

The clue pointing to a role for serotonin in the functioning of the central nervous system came from its discovery in the brain by two British pharmacologists, John Gaddum and Khan A. Hameed. At the time, Gaddum was studying ergot compounds, which are also strong vasoconstrictors.

Ergot is derived from a fungus, *Claviceps purpurea*, that grows on rye. Many of the alkaloids it contains are neurotoxic, and many of them are hallucinogenic: the lysergic acids, the lysergic acid amides, and the ergopeptides.[15]

Ergot causes severe vasoconstriction as well as hallucinations. Gaddum hypothesized that ergot's vasoconstrictive effect on blood vessels would also be true in the brain. He went on to discover that ergot alkaloids counteracted the constrictive action of serotonin on smooth muscle tissue. Gaddum found that lysergic acid, or LSD, was the most potent of the eight ergot alkaloids he examined for their ability to antagonize (that is counteract the function of) serotonin in both rat uteri and rabbit ear preparations. He concluded the psychoactive effects of LSD were in some way related to the way it interacted with serotonin in the brain.[16]

In 1965, the hypothesis that depression was caused by a chemical imbalance was put forward by psychiatrist Joseph Schildkraut, whose research on the biochemical classification of depressive disorders set the stage for an unkillable urban mythology around depression being caused by the disruption of serotonin levels in the brain. Such a disruption, he posited, would result in the failure of electrochemical signal transmission between neurons. Schildkraut's theory flew in the face of existing research. A 1957 paper had already written off the idea entirely. Pharmacologists Bernard Brodie and Parkhurst Shore, working at the US National Institutes of Health, wrote: "If the role of serotonin (or norepinephrine) in brain function is that of a chemical mediator . . . it seems unlikely that the many kinds of mental illnesses could possibly be explained by the single premise of faulty nerve transmission. This seems too easy a solution of the problem."[17]

Rather than shelving the "chemical imbalance" theory, as the two NIH pharmacologists had done almost a decade before, the research and pharmaceutical establishment pursued Schildkraut's hypothesis with a vengeance, publishing paper after paper, desperate to declare a serotonin deficit as the single most determinative factor in depression.

Then, a thread of evidence emerged in the late 1960s implicating serotonin in major depressive disorder: A postmortem study revealed decreased concentrations of serotonin in brains of depressed individuals who had committed suicide, a signature bit of information that sent pharmas and researchers careening down a fateful and specious path where correlation was conveniently mistaken for causation.[18] There could have been several factors causing disruption of serotonin synthesis before death, and there could have been postmortem catabolism immediately afterward.[19] There are, in fact, organ systems and generative processes that continue functioning for a short while following death. Yet any possible factors that could have caused lowered serotonin levels in corpses were summarily ignored.

Like many of their peers, scientists at the pharmaceutical company Eli Lilly followed the growing stampede and pursued the serotonin-deficit theory of depression. They began working on a compound to prevent serotonin reuptake from brain synapses in the early 1970s. Once the reuptake process is halted, the space between neurons is continuously flooded with serotonin, creating a scenario of nonstop electrochemical signaling.

In a normally functioning brain, once a presynaptic neuron has released serotonin into the synaptic gap, it must be removed quickly in order to terminate the signal between the two neurons. A small amount is metabolized by an enzyme, monoamine oxidase, to the corresponding aldehyde. Excess serotonin not taken up by the postsynaptic neuron is reabsorbed by the presynaptic side. SSRIs block this mechanism.

Dismantling the stop button between the two neurons by flooding the space with serotonin, or 5-HT, is theorized to be the therapeutic element of SSRIs: In other words, halting a neurochemical process necessary for balancing signal transmission in the brain was deemed a therapeutic breakthrough. The brain, however, as a homeostatic system designed by evolution to keep itself in neurochemical balance, reacts to this flood of synaptic 5-HT, signaling the presynaptic neurons to fire at a slower rate. Soon, in response, far less serotonin is released into the synapse. The postsynaptic neurons then also must adjust themselves. The corresponding receptors on the postsynaptic side are downregulated—fewer are created by the cells. The reduction in receptor density causes the biochemical interchange in the brain to stop working.

Although this appears to be a definitive thwarting of the drug's action by the brain, a response researchers called "synaptic resilience," another change also occurs, one much more dire in terms of the brain's capacity to rebalance itself neurochemically.

The autoreceptors for serotonin on the presynaptic neurons also decline in number in response to the reduced amount of serotonin in the synapse, thus disabling the feedback mechanism. All the while, serotonin continues to be produced in the brain stem. With no off switch to control the serotonergic system functioning on either side, presynaptic neurons begin to fire at a normal rate again, at least for a while, causing even more serotonin than normal to accumulate in a system where there is no longer a mechanism to remove it.[20] These gyrations in brain chemistry, unsurprisingly, created a great many problems for patients who were given the drug. And it was not as though Eli Lilly was unaware of the problems with its new compound, fluoxetine hydrochloride.

Following some disastrous results of a Phase 3 clinical trial conducted in Germany in the early 1980s, the *Bundesgesundheitsamt* or BGA, the German equivalent of the US Food and Drug Administration (FDA), summarily rejected the company's application for approval for the drug in the German market. The drug, besides providing little or no improvement in patients, caused psychosis, hallucinations, and, in some patients, increased anxiety, agitation, and insomnia. The worst side effects, though, were the suicide attempts and successful suicides: Sixteen attempts were made; two were successful. A German Eli Lilly employee privately calculated the incidence rate of suicides was 5.6 times higher with fluoxetine than another antidepressant drug, imipramine.[21]

In its application for FDA approval, Eli Lilly did its best to hide any adverse events. At least one FDA reviewer, Richard Kapit, worried about its safety.[22] Fluoxetine, Kapit concluded, "may negatively affect patients with depression."

But rather than allow its fanaticism about its new drug to decelerate, Eli Lilly characterized every adverse event, such as suicide, as a symptom of depression itself.

Robert Whitaker, a journalist who has brilliantly gotten up the nostrils of the psychiatric and pharmaceutical establishments through his exhaustive reading and analysis of thousands of scientific papers attempting to prove a biological basis for mental disorders (there is none, as he showed repeatedly in his landmark book, *Anatomy of an Epidemic*), writes, "At least 39 patients treated with fluoxetine had gone psychotic in the short trials. . . . Other side effects included insomnia, nervousness, confusion, dizziness, memory dysfunction, tremors, and impaired motor coordination."[23]

Despite a lack of any real clinical evidence that the drug provided any benefit at all, fluoxetine was approved by the FDA in December of 1987 and was launched to the US market by Eli Lilly in January 1988 under the trade name Prozac.

Prozac turned out to be the most complained-about drug on MedWatch, the FDA's website for post-market, adverse-event reporting. Reports poured in of people committing crimes, killing themselves, and experiencing psychotic depression, mania, abnormal thinking, hallucinations, hostility, confusion, amnesia, convulsions, tremors, and sexual dysfunction. Undeterred, Eli Lilly's marketing machine swung into action. Scientific reports written by doctors with ties to the pharmaceutical company extolled its virtues. At a 1991 hearing convened by the FDA about adverse effects, a panel of citizens who voiced their concerns was outgunned by an advisory panel composed of pharma-aligned physicians who made sure the discussion was limited to presentations that supported Eli Lilly's interests. A Lilly supporter told *The Wall Street Journal* that the entire controversy over the drug was a "complete fiction . . . organized and funded by an anti-psychiatric movement."[24]

By then, the FDA had become nothing more than a turnkey operation for approval of new pharmaceutical drugs. Safety considerations took a back seat to the drug's potential to turn a profit.

In an article in *Prevention and Treatment*, Irving Kirsch described the efficacy data submitted to the FDA between 1987 and 1999 in support of the approval of the six most widely prescribed antidepressants (fluoxetine, paroxetine, sertraline, venlafaxine, nefazodone, and citalopram).

The story is grim.

The FDA requires positive results from at least two controlled clinical trials, but the total number of trials can vary. A memorandum discussing the approval action for citalopram describes two efficacy trials showing a significant difference between drug and placebo. Three others "failed to provide results" confirming the positive findings.[25] For the evaluator, however, this result led him to conclude that "there is clear evidence from more than one adequate and well-controlled clinical investigation that citalopram exerts an antidepressant effect. The size of that effect, and more importantly the clinical value of that effect is not something that can be validly measured. . . . Accordingly, substantial evidence in the present case, as it has in all other evaluations of antidepressant effectiveness, speaks to proof in principle of a product's effectiveness."[26]

The FDA Division of Neuropharmacological Drug Products team leader for psychiatric drug products commented, "While the reasons for negative outcomes are unknown . . . there was substantial placebo response, making it difficult to distinguish drug from placebo." He concluded, "I feel there were sufficient reasons to speculate about the negative outcomes and, therefore, not count these studies against citalopram."[27]

As far as the FDA was concerned, psychotropic drugs for depression did not even need to work, side effects and toxicity be damned. Potential long-term effects were not even mentioned.

PRESCRIBED DRUG DEPENDENCE

In the late 1980s, advertisements for SSRI antidepressants began flooding the media in the United States. New pills could make people feel better than well. Patients were promised that they'd never be blue again and that they would experience only happy, clappy, and chirpy feelings forevermore. Psychiatrist Peter Kramer's 1993 book *Listening to Prozac* announced a new mental health era, the dawn of "cosmetic psychopharmacology." Yet within a decade, it was clear that antidepressants and antianxiety medications were not living up to their hype. Moreover, both patients and doctors were rapidly discovering their downsides, which were terrifying.

Rather than improving, mental health outcomes rapidly deteriorated once SSRI pharmaceutical drugs flooded the market.

Dr. David Healy, professor of psychiatry at Bangor University, North Wales, and consulting psychiatrist at North Wales Department of Psychological Medicine Hergest Unit in Bangor, reviewed records from patients treated at the North Wales Asylum in Denbigh in the 1890s and compared them with records from psychiatric patients treated at the District General Hospital in Bangor during the 1990s. Between 1894 and 1896, there were only 45 people admitted per year. Fifty percent were discharged as "recovered" and another 30 percent as "relieved."[28] Mentally ill inpatients, including psychotic patients, got better over the course of several months to a year and were discharged into their families and into the community. Until the 1990s, mental illnesses, including psychosis, were transient and self-limiting conditions from which patients recovered during a period of anywhere from several months to a year. The latter group (psychotics) averaged only 1.23 hospitalizations in a ten-year period. (That number includes the initial hospitalization).[29] Most went on to live productive lives and did not return.

Now, however, the picture is decidedly different.

In 1996, by contrast, 522 people were admitted to the psychiatric ward in Bangor. Seventy-six percent of these had been there before, part of a large group of patients that cycled regularly through the hospital. Although stays were shorter than in 1896, only 36 percent were discharged as recovered. The patients admitted for a first episode of psychosis in the 1990s averaged 3.96 hospitalizations over the course of ten years—more than three times the number a century earlier.[30] Healy observed that, years ago, some used to recover spontaneously.

But now, rather than waiting to see how people are faring when they first seek treatment, doctors immediately put all patients on medications, creating a situation where doctors run the risk of giving patients chronic problems. Healy is a firm believer in the "watch and wait" method. And, if a treatment isn't doing what it's supposed to do, he stops it. His tactic, unfortunately, is the exception rather than the rule. Most doctors simply switch medications, convinced that if a patient is "failing" one treatment, the answer can only be to change medication or pile another on top of it to combat its side effects, a kind of riff on the motivational technique of hitting the mule over the head with a two-by-four when all the whipping in the world has failed to make it walk forward.

Simply removing the offending medication is rarely the chosen course of action.

More recent studies have revealed a continuation of the troubling trend noted by Healy.

Dr. Michael Hengartner analyzed mental health outcome data from the longitudinal Zurich Cohort Study, a long-range survey instituted by clinicians at the Zurich University Psychiatric Hospital in the late 1970s to assess the prevalence of mental disorders in the general population.[31] Selected in 1978, the study group consisted of a randomly chosen representative sample of 4,547 nineteen- and twenty-year-olds from Zurich, Switzerland. A subgroup of 591 people who were identified as having increased psychopathological distress was selected for a long-term study. Members of the group were interviewed in 1979 and again in 1981, 1986, 1988, 1993, 1999, and 2008, when they were forty-nine and fifty years old.

Over the course of the entire thirty-year observation period, antidepressant use was 6 percent in persons with depression symptoms, 7 percent in those with mild depression, and 22 percent in those with major depression. Independent of severity, and the condition of the participant at the start of the study, antidepressant use was found to predict poorer long-term outcomes in levels of depression and corresponding symptoms. Those with the worst depression symptoms over the long term were suicidal at baseline, which is when the study began.

The most important factor in whether symptoms improve, noted Hengartner, is an effect that has been observed repeatedly in placebo trials.

"Regular contact with the physician is the most important factor in positive outcomes," said Hengartner when I spoke to him. "The active ingredient is human contact."

But modern psychiatry does not care to see it that way. They'd prefer to take a punt in favor of the pharmaceutical companies and continue with biochemical interventions, long-term study results be damned.

People who have been taking these medications long term and have suffered terrible consequences are now beginning to fight back against medical and psychiatric guild systems that, far from helping, are making them sicker. In the United States, Britain, Norway, and a growing number of other countries, groups have formed to address the medical and mental health issues that long-term use of psychotropic medications regimens have caused.

Adele Framer, founder of the website SurvivingAntidepressants.org, a comprehensive online peer-support website for those who have tried or who are trying to taper off psychiatric drugs, recounts an unfortunately common story.[32] At the age of fifty, she was prescribed ten milligrams of the SSRI paroxetine for treatment of work-related stress. She rapidly developed numerous symptoms, including psychological and sexual numbing. She tried to switch to escitalopram, which she describes as disastrous. She sought advice from an outpatient psychiatric clinic and, receiving none, tapered herself off paroxetine over the course of a few weeks.

Once off paroxetine, Framer experienced a horrific range of symptoms: hypomania, sweating, and "brain zaps"—the feeling that electricity is being shot through the brain. As time passed, she underwent feelings of depersonalization, insomnia, light and heat intolerance, indigestion, palpitations, unease, spontaneous crying spells, attacks of sheer terror, and sudden plunges into black holes of pure dread. She concluded this was not a relapse. She spent hours searching journal articles about antidepressant withdrawal syndrome. Psychiatrists refused her request for reinstatement of paroxetine, despite the many articles indicating this was the appropriate course of action.

Many patients, realizing it's the drug that's making them sick, are dismissed outright by their psychiatrists. Writing on the website "Mad in America," prescribed-psychiatric-drug survivor Rose Yesha notes:

> [Psychiatrists] see injured patients as a liability, individuals which may present them with further problems down the line. Furthermore, they may see injured patients as a threat to their profession: if they are to admit that psychiatric medications can and do cause harm, what would that mean for the future of their careers?[33]

In no other specialty, she writes, would iatrogenically injured patients be gaslighted and told that their new symptoms are the result of another underlying pathology.

IS IT TIME TO ABOLISH PSYCHIATRY?

Earlier in this chapter, I wrote about the *DSM*, a book that turned the notion of mental health squarely on its head. I'm closing the chapter with a book I wish offered a thoroughly vetted road map on how to repair our current mental health crisis, complete with a suggested infrastructure plan and projected budget. Alas, not so.

Instead, the book, penned by Dr. Thomas Insel, America's most influential mental health expert, is a *faux* apologia, a mélange of gaslighting and humble brag. Insel, who ran the National Institute of Mental Health (NIMH) from 2002 until 2015—the longest-serving director in the agency's history—could not have done less to improve mental health outcomes in the United States. And he spent over $22 billion of public funds doing it.

Insel's thirteen-year tenure in his self-proclaimed role as "America's psychiatrist" was noteworthy not for the progress he made in relieving suffering—the long-forgotten original charter of the medical profession—but rather for his expensive pursuit of biomedical research agendas, ignoring the public he was supposed to be serving.

In a review of Insel's recent book, *Healing: Our Path from Mental Illness to Mental Health*, on the website Mad in America, Andrew Scull—a British-born sociologist who studies the social history of medicine and the history of psychiatry—provides background about how present-day NIMH priorities developed:

> For the first three decades of its existence, the new institute pursued an eclectic approach to the problems posed by major mental illness, funding social and behavioral

research alongside biological and pharmacological studies. That broad-spectrum approach was abruptly abandoned under Reagan's presidency. Research that suggested connections between mental illness and social factors was distinctly unwelcome politically, and faced with threats to the organization's funding, the leaders of NIMH embraced a research agenda that focused narrowly on biological psychiatry.[34]

Rather than trying to maintain or at least nod at what one president of the American Psychiatric Association characterized as a bio-psycho-social approach to the problem of mental illness, Insel decapitated the psycho-social pursuit. With the so-called Research Domain Criteria (RDoC), Insel introduced an alternative approach for research: *conceptualizing all mental illnesses as brain disorders,* thereby reducing the agency's approach to a feckless pursuit of genetic and neurochemical biomarkers as determinants of mental illness. *In other words, the NIMH would henceforth pick up where the pharmaceutical industry and the DSM left off.*

According to the new axiom, reactive, traumatic, and environmental causes of mental illness and emotional disorders do not exist. There would henceforth be no such thing as mental illness stemming from adverse childhood events, abuse, poverty, violence, foul air, hunger, homelessness, or lack of education. No emotional, cognitive, or behavior change would be attributable to any circumstance whatsoever in the outside world, whether caused by war, violence, the COVID-19 pandemic, or the climate crisis.

Everything about your response or my response to a toxic world was not a problem with the world. Rather, according to the RDoC, the problem was caused by something intrinsically wrong with our very own brains.

And yet, none of the costly and idiotic research activity under Insel's governance produced a single outcome yielding any benefit at all to clinical medicine.

Insel's lack of concern toward ordinary humans was borne out by the numbers. During his very long time in his government post, US suicide rates skyrocketed. In 2008, suicide ranked as the tenth leading cause of death for all ages in the United States according to CDC data. In 2016—a year after Insel's departure—suicide became the second leading cause of death among those aged ten to thirty-four (yes, ten years of age) and the fourth leading cause among those aged thirty-five to fifty-four. The number of people on government disability due to mood disorders jumped from a bit over 880,000 in 2002 to over 2 million in 2013.[35]

In his introduction to the book, whose fulsome descriptions of his government-service duties suggest he's on the short list for a sainthood, Insel displayed a false humility about his time in government.

"I should have been able to bend the curves for death and disability. But I didn't. Because I misunderstood the problem. Or maybe it's more accurate to say that the problem I was solving by supporting brilliant scientists and dedicated clinicians was not the problem that faced nearly fifteen million Americans living with serious mental illness," he said.[36]

In a 2017 interview in *Wired* magazine, Insel said, "I spent thirteen years at NIMH really pushing on the neuroscience and genetics of mental disorders. . . . I don't think we moved the needle in reducing suicide, reducing hospitalizations, improving recovery for the tens of millions of people who have mental illness. I hold myself accountable for that."[37]

His were crocodile tears.

Having spent thirteen years squandering public funds and the public trust, Insel declared the intention to figure out why, in light of a dramatic jump in the number of people taking psychiatric drugs and receiving outpatient care, disability numbers were rising and the mentally ill were dying fifteen to thirty years earlier than the general population.

Evidently, he did not read the scientific literature.

In 2015, after being asked during an interview for the film *Letters from Generation RX* about the "science of psychiatric drugs," Insel said that *Anatomy of an Epidemic* made an important point: "If you increase the use of your medication [in other areas of medicine] twofold, threefold, sixfold, you will see—we have seen, reductions in morbidity and mortality." This, he said, had not been the case since the "enormous increase in the use of antidepressants, antipsychotics, and other neuroleptic or psychotropic medication, which is that broad class, over the last two to three decades."[38]

With the publication of Insel's own book, he recanted this position and summarily dismissed the evidence borne out by hundreds of studies and public data showing psychotropic medical interventions are making things worse rather than better as "a conspiracy theory."

In an essay titled "Thomas Insel Makes a Case for Abolishing Psychiatry," on Mad in America, Robert Whitaker, the website's publisher, writes:

> He assures readers that such medications are necessary. . . .
> The blame for the poor outcomes, it seems, falls on society
> for not investing in necessary social supports and on patients
> who fail to take their drugs and stay engaged in treatment.
>
> There is nothing in that narrative that could be expected
> to harm psychiatry's guild interests or pharmaceutical
> interests.[39]

Insel's book describes how he discovered what he found to be a brilliant revelation into healing from a psychiatrist toiling away on Los Angeles's Skid Row. People need more than just medicine, the doctor told him, they need "people, place, and purpose," or the "three Ps." By itself, the insight is hardly original and something every person interested in public health, human bonds, and the integrity of the social fabric knows: People need community, a sense of belonging, and a sense of mission in order to both survive and thrive.

Insel, though, despite his new knowledge, could not abandon his insistence that current treatments work, be they psychiatric drugs, electroconvulsive therapy, ketamine infusions—or maybe, if he'd been around 125 years or so ago, nasal cavity surgery? All these invasive procedures and pharmaceutical therapies *must work*. Why ever should anyone believe this in the face of overwhelming evidence to the contrary?

Insel continues to advocate zealously for medical and pharmaceutical interventions while reams of data pile up against them. And yet, as Whitaker points out, in a book of over three hundred pages, "What is notable is that he didn't cite a single study that told of psychiatric drugs providing a long-term benefit."

He didn't because there isn't one.

I occasionally speak to a retired brigadier general psychiatrist and medical ethicist who served as an advisor to the Joint Chiefs of Staff and other senior Department of Defense officials during the Obama administration. During that time, he advocated for psychological health care for veterans and for treating veterans for the effects of blast concussions. He has worked with torture survivors at Guantanamo. He is the only retired military general and physician to speak out publicly against torture and the involvement of health care practitioners in torture. His mission is clearly and overwhelmingly to relieve human suffering. He is well acquainted with the bureaucratic brass at the US Department of Health and Human Services.

He witnessed Insel in action as Insel cruised around and through government organizations. He described Insel to me as "a textbook sociopath" who "has perfected the art of spending other people's money to enrich himself. Then when he's used up the goods, his sociopathy makes it easy for him to fail upward: He simply moves on to the next opportunity, the next person or institution he can exploit for his own gain."

Now having declared the "three Ps" as the way forward, Insel made sure he was not the one responsible for implementing them. He'd already squandered the money in the public coffers on his famously useless RDoC junket. That ship already sailed. Dealing with ordinary people and their needs was a bridge too far. Besides, it would not profit him in the slightest.

Instead, Insel discovered the beauty of the Silicon Valley startup. In 2017, Insel joined a company called Mindstrong that employed an all-new *new* idea (Silicon Valley produces one every few hours) called "digital phenotyping" as a diagnostic tool. By combining data from electronic medical records with tracking apps to record how people use their gadgets, Mindstrong theorized the predictive possibilities of studying individual keyboard-usage patterns would become a gold mine of mental health data just waiting to be exploited.

Now, even keystrokes can be indicators of mental illness. The very idea is terrifying. Imagine being in a bad mood one day or drinking too much coffee and banging away on your Facebook account too vigorously. Your bad day could be electronically metastasized into a full-blown diagnosis of schizophrenia.

Insel apparently would not dream of asking patients what they actually need or engage in the creation of livable communities designed to improve human connection and mental health outcomes. He would rather use cell phones as surveillance tools to spy on the daily thoughts and feelings of ordinary people obsessively doomscrolling on Twitter, people who can't connect with one another despite being wired to computational systems 24-7.

Surveillance capitalism is the new "new" thing in predictive behavioral tools. Now we have spyware as medicine. More diagnoses to name, more pills to dispense. Pills won't be the only behavioral-management tool of the future. There are already intracranial implants, designed to zap your brain into submission when your cell phone detects an aberration.[40] Perhaps we should just be honest and call them a cure for "thought crimes."

Twenty-two billion dollars and thirteen years later, one would have hoped America's erstwhile psychiatrist would finally grok that naming a specious diagnosis and placing it inside the head of an individual isn't an answer and has nothing to do with healing anything. Yet, to "America's psychiatrist," this is a nonissue. He's doing well, thank you very much.

Insel is not unlike many of the psychiatrists I've met over the years. He satisfies his ego by telling himself and those around him the single reason he's doing well is because he is doing good. His gift for gaslighting is a signature feature of psychiatric medicine—What is it they do, actually?—while the long con, feeding his voracious appetite for fame, fortune, and professional cred, continues.

CHAPTER 5

THE SHATTERING

M y senior year in college, I moved from a group house on campus to a small house with two roommates, my best friend in college, S, and a childhood friend who transferred to Stanford after a year at an East Coast school. He and I had spent many hours of our childhood and teenage years together. Despite our friendship, I never confided in him. A mama's boy, he had always been a people pleaser, obsessed with status and appearances, and deeply conflicted about women. I knew even as a child I could never trust him to take my part.

I had been accepted to the Humanities Honors program as a junior. The demands were ferocious and included reading and writing proficiency in at least two foreign languages. Even though I studied hard, I believed when I started college I would likely not remain after my sophomore year. I had a boyfriend in Norway, a young man I'd met when I worked there for a long summer when I was eighteen, part of a gap-year trip I made after I finished high school. I figured I'd go back to Norway and marry him, eventually. Although I visited him, I did not drop out of college or set a date for my return. At some point, he gave up on me and met someone else.

Only then did I conclude I should probably find a way to determine the path of my own life. If I were to graduate with honors, I'd at least have something to show for myself when managing in the outside world. It did not occur to me to apply for internships. I did not know what they were and did not have anyone to guide me. My energy was exhausted by the demands of trying to navigate the excruciating and poisonous dynamics of my family of origin. I realized years on how determined my parents were to control the minds of family members in order to protect themselves from any revelation about who they really were. I had no concept of how one planned one's future. After a brief run at premed courses in my freshman year, thinking vet school might be an option, I concluded that for me medicine was a nonstarter.

In the spring, a visiting professor from Germany, Professor F, invited me to attend a party with him, a *Faschingsball*—like a Carnival party—thrown by the German Studies department.

I knew F because I had stayed with his family in Berlin during a two-month course in German during my gap year. They were an academic family, with four children several years younger than my siblings and me. I agreed to attend with him, despite a terrible sinus infection. I did not own anything resembling an evening gown. Eventually I found a long, loose-fitting maroon rayon dress and a pair of sandals. Hardly evening attire but what I could afford.

F had no wheels—he was only in residence for a few months—so I agreed to borrow a car from my parents for the evening. Afterward, I would return the car to my parents' house, and one of my roommates would come and collect me from there.

I felt awkward the moment we arrived at the party. I was embarrassed being seen with this man who was old enough to be my father. My sinus pain was so severe it radiated to my jaw, rendering me incapable of either eating or drinking. I watched the other guests, captivated by the movements of a lissome woman in a diaphanous frock decorated with raised appliqué embroidery as she frolicked on the dance floor, glass lifted to her lips, her *Kasper Nase* rolling upward as she quaffed champagne from the tall flute.

I danced one dance, to be polite.

We left early, and I drove F back to the house where he was staying, not far from my parents' home. I halted the car in front of his driveway, said good night, and waited for him to exit. Then he threw himself on top of me, grabbed my breasts, and thrust his tongue at my mouth. I pulled away, shoved my door open, and leaped out. I stood in the road, shaking. I told him to get out. At first, he did not budge. I repeated myself, adding that I had to return the car. He opened the door and removed himself a bit too casually from the passenger's side. I jumped back in the car and sped off. I arrived at my parents' house, intending to leave the car and call my roommate to come fetch me. Hearing me at the front door, my mother appeared at the top of the stairs, drunk.

"How was the party?" She puffed a cigarette.

"I don't want to talk about it," I replied.

"It must have been fun."

"F jumped me," I said. Feeling nauseated, I lay down in the hallway.

My mother was silent for a few moments. I heard her feet descending the staircase. She stopped beside me and stood over me.

In a tone of mild distaste, she said, "You're acting like a rape victim."

I half expected her to shove at me with her toe.

I raised myself from the floor, stood up unsteadily, and walked past her up the stairs, depositing the keys on the dining room table. I called my roommate, S, and went out again to wait at the top of the driveway until she arrived.

Looking back, all the signals were there. In Berlin, he had insisted on taking me to the opera and to the symphony as part of my so-called education. His wife preferred not to go. On these soirees, he made what I later recognized as overtly salacious comments. Thoroughly brainwashed and trained not to see predatory behavior for what it was, I brushed these verbal degradations aside as lighthearted jest.

Gaslighting myself was a conditioned response. The wife, for her part, an intelligent, educated woman who had studied literature, had given up on herself. She devoted her life to the children and the tasks of a homemaker. She smoked incessantly. She pulled bottles of *Sekt* out of the cellar and opened a box of cordial cherries, which she consumed over the course of the evening. She helped me with my German, ploughing through novels of my choosing, all of which were far beyond my skill level at the time. She was one of the kindest people I had ever met and I developed a real attachment to her.

I am unable to discern, looking back, to what degree she was kidding herself about her husband.

On the way home, I told S what happened. As a woman from the Middle East, the daughter of a Saudi father and an American mother who spent her childhood in Beirut and Cairo, she was familiar with acts of misogyny.

I did not have a lot of time to spend on my emotional distress. It was spring, and I had a thesis to write. Then a few weeks later, the phone rang. The German-accented voice did not identify himself, rather asked me to guess who it was. I hung up.

At the time of the incident, my roommates and I had been living in the house in Redwood City for only a few weeks. I had never given Professor F my phone number. He had conveyed his invitation to the ball through my parents, and when I responded, I was at their home. I had known instinctively not to give him my contact information.

I rang my mother and asked if she had given him the number. She was silent for a moment.

"No," she said.

"Who did?"

"Your father," she said.

"Does he know what happened?"

She paused, inhaling a cigarette. "Yes," she said.

"And what did you say?"

She said nothing. Then, she said, "If you're upset, maybe you should talk to Cleo."

Cleo was a social worker, one of my mother's few friends. While I did not dislike her—she was a kind woman by nature—she was part of the same cabal.

In her living room a few evenings later, she regarded me sympathetically.

"Do you think your father might have thought he was calling to apologize?" she asked.

"No," I said.

"What then?"

The last thing she would want to hear was about how little my father valued his daughters—particularly me—and how he identified with predators. I thanked her for her time and departed.

On a cellular level, I understood my father's actions the way most targets of predators do, when we're able to be honest with ourselves. Providing Professor F my phone number was a nod and fist bump, predator to predator. A gesture of tribal signaling. They know the thoughts of each other's minds the way con men do; the same detection facility leads wolves to each other's hunting grounds.

Viewed through the lens of my father's narcissism, this man did my father a favor. His not-so-secret worry about his daughters' desirability to males could be eased a bit. That I'd had boyfriends did not register. I hadn't revealed my plan to marry my Norwegian beau to my parents. My chosen partners were not right for my father's taste. They were not my father's kind. The predator kind.

A few weeks later, a card addressed to me in characteristic *Sütterlinschrift* arrived in the mail at our Redwood City house. I threw it away without opening it.

No sane man gives his child's coordinates to her attacker. The impulse of a sane man is to go tear out the throat of anyone who tries to harm his flesh and blood.

One friend, when I told him what happened, declared he would go to the guy's office and beat the shit out of him. He'd recently been admitted to law school. I refused to allow him to do it. I did not want him to ruin his career.

Reasoning like this could not have been further from my father's nature. Rather, my father was a man who, a bit over a decade prior, had taken my siblings and me to the Red Light District in Amsterdam, where topless, thong-clad prostitutes undulated in red-neon-lit Perspex display windows.

On spying us walking down the street, one woman standing in a doorway screamed, "What are you doing here with these children? What kind of parent are you? Take them home, you motherfucker."

My father waved her off.

At the end of the migraine-riven, sleep-deprived term, I completed my honor's thesis, earning the highest honors available. Comically, my academic accolades were a point of some envy to friends of my sisters, all recent Radcliffe graduates, one of whom sent me a "congratulations, graduate" card.

After the school-wide commencement ceremony in the amphitheater, I joined my fellow editor from the literary magazine at the English Department's degree-conferring ceremony, mistakenly assuming my awards ceremony was to take place there. I soon realized I was in the wrong place, perhaps, in hindsight, an error with a purpose, a premonition about what was about to come to pass. A professor directed me to another location in the quad.

By the time I arrived where I was supposed to be, the program was already well underway. I ensconced myself among a group of classmates at the back of the crowd. Then, my attention was drawn to the podium: my father ascending the steps to the makeshift stage. A classmate beside me recognized me.

"Erica, they've already called your name," she said. "You should go up. Is that your father?"

"Yes," I replied. I felt sick. "I think they thought I wasn't here, so he's going to take it for me."

"No, no," she said. "Go up."

At that moment, the dean spied me in the crowd and waved. I was mortified. Pushed gently forward by classmates, I made my way to the podium. I could see my father holding my diploma in his hand. The dean had handed it to him.

Stanford, unbeknownst to me, had a bizarre tradition of encouraging faculty whose children attend the school to bestow diplomas on their hapless offspring, as though, after all these hours and years and sweat, the honors had something to do with them. And there was my father, who had given my phone number and address to the man who had assaulted me not three months prior, about to hand me my diploma.

At the podium, I numbly shook the dean's hand and took the diploma from my father without making eye contact. When he tried to grasp my hand in his, I pulled away and dashed back down to the back of the gathering.

It was as though my father was graduating, earning at my expense honors higher than he himself had ever achieved. I had done something wrong, and the diploma belonged to him, not to me. With this gesture, my shame and terror about being my parents' daughter began to metastasize. A man who had nothing to offer the world, when one examined it—a fact that his job at a prestigious institution disguised for him—one moment devalued my life so thoroughly he gave my phone number to my assailant and, at the next, stole the limelight of my graduation with highest honors from me. I wanted nothing to do with him, but I made the error of having been born with gifts he envied. A man who never ceased moaning about how he was victimized by his circumstances was going to cash in on my God-given talent.

Not long after, I put a match to my Stanford diploma and burned it in a wastebasket.

Soon after graduation, I set off for England. I had obtained a UK work permit, courtesy of a government program available to recent US college graduates.

For a few weeks, I stayed in a London suburb at the home of a friend from high school. I went looking for work. I interviewed at several publishing houses. Then I began to feel poorly. Exhausted all the time, I could barely get out of bed. I began vomiting. Although I was parked in my friend's bedroom, she was not living at home but had her own flat with a friend. As an unwell person spending entirely too much time in a darkened room, I knew I was outstaying my welcome at her parents' house. I found a cheap hotel room near St. Pancras station. I spent days in and out of bed, vomiting. When I finally managed to rouse myself enough to go out, I knew I had no choice but to return to California. I had nowhere else to go.

My parents were none too happy to see me. Because they had rented all of the children's bedrooms to Stanford students, except my old room—my grandmother was using it—I stayed in a family room off the dining room. The practice of renting our rooms as a dormitory was my parents' riposte to their children for having inconvenienced them. They were determined to recoup their investment in having raised us. Except for my sister D, the house was not ours. Her room remained vacant for a time in case she wanted to return home.

To underscore how deeply my parents felt burdened by my presence, they charged me rent and required I pay for my food as well as cook at least one meal a week for them and my grandmother.

I soon found two jobs: working as a technical writer for a pharmaceutical startup and as a tutor. I bought a car and commuted between one and the other, clocking one hundred miles a day.

Staying with my parents was the stupidest thing I could have done. D had stayed with them the year she'd graduated from college before she started medical school, ostensibly to save money. On some level, I felt I was entitled to the same treatment. I refused to accept the truth about how little regard they had for me or my life. I resumed a relationship with a boyfriend I'd been seeing before I left, a young Chinese American man in his senior year of college.

I spent as much time as possible when not at work at the houses of friends.

But something was really wrong. While still in England, I visited a doctor who diagnosed me with "traveler's illness" and suggested I change my diet to something blander. Once in California, I went to a doctor my parents used. He suggested I was suffering from fatigue. Or it was something I ate. He took a stool sample. No one asked about my menstrual cycle or suggested a pregnancy test.

My periods had been irregular since they started in my mid-teens. I was an obsessive dieter and exerciser. I ran several times a week. I swam. I rode my bicycle miles and miles: to the beach and then to a barn in the foothills to take riding lessons. All the dieting and exercise meant I was extremely thin. My periods often stopped altogether for months at a time. Because I was mostly amenorrheic, I was never very careful about birth control. I became even less so after I graduated college. I felt nothing belonged to me, not my life, not my body, not my mind, not even my degree. My parents would take credit for my achievements, and the only thing I could count on was their piling on more abuse to any degradation or misfortune that came my way.

One night, my boyfriend awakened from a dream, shaken. He had dreamed about a baby alone someplace in a street or a field, uncared for and vulnerable. Rats were chewing at its head. He'd commented once or twice that my body had changed. I refused to see it. He even told me one day he thought he felt a head when he had his hand on my belly.

The dream made my blood run cold. I jumped out of bed and ran into the bathroom. In the mirror, the front of my nightgown was wet, streaked with yellowish, pinkish fluid. I pulled it off and stared. I knew nothing at all about pregnancy. I could not have recited the telltale signs. I'd never read about or been informed of the symptoms. But there in the mirror in front of me was the reality of my now-pregnant body—enlarged breasts where before there practically were none, a faint brown stripe from my pubis to my navel, liquid leaking from my nipples. And my belly. My clothes no longer fit the way they used to, and there were trousers that couldn't zip up, but I was so thin, I dismissed the bulge as some kind of localized weight gain.

I was trained by my parents to believe my not feeling well, whether physically or mentally or emotionally, was yet another indication that I was poorly wrought. I was ever wrong and at fault, and *there was something fundamentally abhorrently wrong with the entirety of my being.* I had long since become so afraid of calling their attention to my fundamental badness and being punished for it, I suppressed any sign or symptom of weakness, including and especially illness. Letting on that I was suffering or incapacitated—as I frequently was with migraines—was at best dismissed as malingering. At worst, I was punished.

On a ski trip in my teens, I was injured in a fall. It was late morning, and on a particularly narrow turn on a steep trail, I caught an edge on the downward side, torquing my knee joint. Losing my balance, I slid off into the deep snow below the slope. My binding released and the ski skidded off into some trees below me. I struggled to right myself in several feet of powder, but blinding pain in my left leg halted me. Then my father appeared on the trail above me. He stopped and asked what was wrong, leaning on his poles. I told him I'd hurt my leg. He sidestepped down the slope a bit, tamped a flat space in the snow beside him with his skis, and ordered me to get up. When I couldn't, he shoved his pole into my face and told me to grasp the basket, which I obediently did. He yanked. Pain shot through my leg, and I cried out. Unable to right myself, I fell back.

"Get up," he ordered.

I replied that I couldn't.

"You're a fucking pain in the ass," he said. "You want to lie there, lie there. I just hope I don't have you around my neck when you're twenty-one."

Then he skied off. Fortunately, a skier glided by a few minutes later and, seeing me, stopped and asked me if I was okay. I was not. My leg was injured. Concerned, he said he'd go find the ski patrol. Another skier who happened along volunteered to stay with me until the ski patrol arrived. After about twenty minutes, two ski patrols arrived with a sledge. They maneuvered themselves around me, removed my remaining ski, lifted me into the sledge, and strapped me down, packing a thermal blanket around me for good measure. They retrieved the loose ski. The patrol who led the descent could not take it on board that I, a minor, had been skiing with a parent who knew I was injured and yet the parent was not there. I had no plausible explanation.

Once deposited at the first aid station, I was given something for the pain, and the nurse made a splint. Another girl who had been brought in with a broken arm was tended solicitously by her parents. Seeing me lying in the neighboring cot, the mother asked me if I was okay, if someone was coming to get me. I said I didn't know. They spoke to the nurse, who told her my father had not been located. I overheard them giving her their address. They lived in San Francisco on Divisadero Street. They asked if someone was going to take me home, or if they could help locate my parents. I wished I could go home with them to Divisadero Street, where they would look after me the way they looked after their own child. Then they left with their daughter, her arm in a sling, wishing for me to be able to go home soon. I wanted to die.

Several hours later, after the last run was announced and the lifts were closed, my father showed up to take me back to the cabin my parents had rented, where my mother had spent the day. I have no recollection of where my siblings were or what they were doing.

A four-hour drive later, back at my parents' house, my mother took me to an emergency room. A young doctor ordered X-rays. In the exam room, he prodded on my patella and twisted my knee joint. I gritted my teeth and tried not to make a sound, though the pain was acute. He regarded me with disbelief.

"Doesn't it hurt?" he demanded.

I nodded, tears running down my face.

"Then why aren't you yelling?" he said. "A football player with this injury would be screaming bloody murder by now."

I started to cry then, wiping my nose on my sleeve. He shook his head and told me and my mother I had "the football player's injury," a torn anterior cruciate ligament. I would need surgery. A cast was put on my leg. He'd do more X-rays in a few weeks.

Back home my father, on hearing the news, declared it was bullshit. There was going to be no surgery. I never skied again.

The night I realized I was pregnant, the fact of my disassociation from my body presented itself to me full-blown and obdurate as bright sunlight on a cloudless day. I did not live in my own body. I was disembodied. I knew the body in the mirror was mine—rather it was a body I could not escape from—but I had no ability to apprehend its physical realities, much less interpret them appropriately. I felt things, to be sure. Since my teens, I had suffered from terrible migraines, which went undiagnosed until a teacher in college insisted I be seen and worked up by a neurologist. My headaches often sent my parents into a rage.

On more than one occasion in my teens, when she heard from my sister that I hadn't gotten out of bed, my mother burst into my bedroom, threw back the covers I'd pulled over my head to block the light, grabbed any available limb, and dragged me onto the floor. In college, they were so severe I lost several days per week to them, particularly my freshman and sophomore years. By my junior year, I'd accumulated so many incompletes I had to stop out for a semester to catch up. I finessed the leave of absence somehow without my parents' knowledge.

Yet none of the emotional or physical torment imposed by my parents' violence mapped coherently onto a rational or comprehending mind. My emotional gyroscope had been dismantled, severed from a proprioceptive body through years of abuse. It was as though my body belonged to a world I once knew existed or believed existed but which had lost its geography. There were no borders; there were no latitude or longitude lines. There was no equator. There were no countries and no pathways around the countryside. My head was somewhere, and my body? It was the incarnation of my "badness," so I had to despise it; it was the locus of my parents' abuse, so I willed it out of existence. I denied my very being in order to survive.

It was years before I understood the medical and emotional sequelae of the abuse. By then, the only thing I knew was I desperately needed to get away from the perpetrators.

But I did not know how to do it.

In the morning, I called my friend S, who was still finishing college. Three years before, she had undergone an illegal abortion in Cairo. She had summoned me to be with her and sent me a ticket for a flight from Bonn, where I was studying at the time.

Now, a few years on, here we were. My abortion would be legal, but far more complicated because I was much further along.

Our first phone call was to Planned Parenthood in Santa Clara. There, a simple test confirmed the pregnancy. They also let it be known I was very far along, over five months by their estimate. They weren't sure I would be able to get an abortion at all. They were certain I couldn't obtain one at their clinic, because they performed abortions only within the first trimester. That I had poor recall of my last period—I guessed the previous August, and it was now January—did not bode well. Because gestation term is determined by fetal head circumference, I needed an ultrasound.

A transvaginal ultrasound placed the fetus at about twenty-two weeks. The nurse at the clinic wanted to make sure I understood that an abortion after twenty-four weeks was illegal in the state of California.

"*Illegal,*" she hissed as she penned numbers on a paper. To obtain a second-trimester abortion I would have to go to a hospital in Oakland, where they were performed as an inpatient procedure.

My emotional state vacillated between panic and numbness. The father wanted me to have the baby. He lost no time contacting an uncle in Taiwan, who offered to take the newborn until I was ready to have it, or perhaps until the father and I were ready to take it. Out of the question for me. I could only imagine what a nightmare trying to extract a baby from an extended Taiwanese family might be once I agreed to relinquish it, especially if I had to travel to Taiwan to get it back. Equally out of the question was my having the child and raising it myself, a possibility my mother posed to me upon learning the news. She claimed she knew all along I was pregnant, although she hadn't said anything. She made up for her muteness a few weeks after the abortion with sentences emerging in a full-blown drunken torrent: "You're a slut, you're irresponsible, you're everyone's worst nightmare, your life is a disaster."

And on. The fact was, my mother liked babies, while they were babies. I believe she would have liked another baby in her life, another little creature with whose life she could tamper. Another unwitting creature whose soul she could destroy.

At the time I underwent the abortion, terror of what would happen to me and a baby belonging to me at the hands of my parents outweighed any other consideration. A zoetrope of scenes replayed in my mind continuously. My parents would find fault with everything I did. They would gaslight me into buying into a belief I was an incompetent mother. They would have me declared unfit for motherhood. They'd have the baby taken from me and would then go to court to obtain legal custody. They'd extract the baby from the father if he tried to claim it. I would be consigned to Nuts on Basement, the Stanford hospital wing located in the basement of the old Hoover Pavilion that was dedicated to younger female psychiatric inpatients. NOB, as it was officially known, existed for the sole purpose of incarcerating young women who could conveniently be labeled as mentally ill. Most of them weren't. They were mostly young women whose families were so toxic and so deadly that the women reacted physically, or emotionally, or rebelled, or ran away.

I knew two girls from Lathrop Drive who had ended up in NOB. Rachel, who coined the Nuts sobriquet, spent a considerable amount of time there. She was an immensely talented young artist, the daughter of a Stanford mathematician. The family lived around the corner. Her sister, J, was in my elementary school class. Their mother's narcissism rivaled that of my father. Rachel's mother envied Rachel's artistic aptitude to the point of distraction.

And there was B, who was a year younger than I. B's family lived in a yellow stucco house next door to my parents. B's father was a professor at Stanford Law School. B became pregnant when she was thirteen years old. When confronted by a high school counselor who demanded to know who the father was, B replied that it was her father. She was promptly remanded to NOB. When she was released a few months later, she didn't return home but went to live someplace else. I don't know what became of the pregnancy.

Rachel did not live at home again either. Rachel created a citadel around her artwork and her life to protect herself from her mother. She died of breast cancer a few years after my sister Andrea's death.

A second-trimester abortion in 1979 in California cost $400 cash and had to take place in a hospital. My boyfriend and I both worked, so the cash was the least of our problems. I would be admitted to the hospital in Oakland overnight. My mother, S, and my boyfriend each wanted to drive me over. In the end, it was the three of them. My mother's demeanor was true to character: preposterous, given the situation at hand, and emotionally unhinged. My boyfriend, not wanting to speak, was politely monosyllabic when my mother addressed him. She tried to engage S in light chitchat about her studies. She made merry and lighthearted comments about the outing. None of us had the courage to tell her to shut up.

Once at the hospital, the procedure was explained: Amniotic fluid would be extracted, saline would be injected, labor would be induced. When I asked what part of the procedure would actually kill the baby, I was instructed sternly by a nurse, "We do not talk about babies, here. We say 'fetus' and 'terminate its growth.'"

My three guests watched while an intravenous line was started. I received a continuous infusion of Pitocin to induce labor. I lay in the bed and waited. When the first cramp arrived, shocking and otherworldly, it was so sudden and severe I cried out in pain, which was very unlike me. The three of them milled around, my mother issuing orders to "breathe." I found their presence intolerable. I wanted them to leave (my mother and my boyfriend; actually, I'd have preferred S stayed) but I could not tell them. I want to scream, *Get out, get out, get the fuck out, get away from me!* But even in that state, I was afraid of what my mother might do if I told her to leave. I feared she would be sufficiently displeased and I'd be punished a few days later for having needs of my own that outweighed hers. Even in this most dire of scenarios, my first thought was how to avoid her rage. I pressed the nurse's buzzer. The nurse entered and perceptively observed my agitation. She asked the three of them to step out and asked me what she could do for me. I told her I was in pain. She did not offer any pain medication.

"It's going to be painful, that's going to be part of it," she said. Then, she said, "I think your mother and your boyfriend and your friend are making things worse for you. Do you want me to ask them to leave?"

I nodded, unequivocally yes. She stepped out. In the hall, I heard her telling them to go home. They'd be called in the morning, when it was time to come fetch me.

Shortly thereafter, the contractions became regular. I began to vomit—and vomit and vomit. The room was kept dark, the lights turned off, blinds drawn. Now and then a nurse entered, looked at the Pitocin bottle, once or twice stuck fingers up my vagina to see how far my cervix was dilated.

Sixteen hours or so later, the fetus emerged. I did not sit up to look at it. I did not want to know anything about this nonbeing. I called the nurse, who prodded on my belly until the placenta came out. Then she folded up the pads underneath me and carried off the remains.

Even now, finding a word to use for what is left of the not-living-yet incarnate form following an abortion is almost impossible. Detritus. Biological material. Thing. Nonlife. Never was.

Perhaps this described me: person who might have been someone but never was and now never would be. That would be my punishment forevermore—never being able to bring anything worth having into the world. Exhausted, I fell asleep.

I spent many years believing I would go to hell, if there was one, yet I cannot think of any alternative decision I could have made at the time that would not have caused me more suffering than I probably could have withstood. I would have had an accident or committed suicide.

The pregnancy and the abortion were the events that finally shattered the iron fortification I spent twenty years building. It forced my dissociated state into my field of vision. From that day forward, I knew something was really, really wrong. A person who did not know she was five months pregnant was missing something. I knew I had to change something, and I would have to climb back into my own body to do it. And to do that, it was essential that I escape from my family of origin, something at the time I had no idea how to do.

The pregnancy also turned out to be my only viable pregnancy. I had a miscarriage in my late thirties, and that was it. Between the endometriosis and an autoimmune disorder, my reproductive life was over. When, in my early forties, it became necessary for me to undergo a hysterectomy—the final nail in the coffin for biological motherhood—a new age but very spiritual woman I know in North Fork, where I lived when I was married, encouraged me to reframe the abortion. She herself had four grown children. One son had stopped speaking to her years before. She insisted on referring to the fetus as a baby. She claimed she could see him. He was a spiritual, nonmaterial being, a little boy.

"I can see his little penis dangling," she said.

Her interpretation was that the baby was an angelic spirit, who had come to me with a message about my life. This was his sole reason for having been conceived, to force me to see, by whatever means possible, that my life was in danger, and I needed to change it. I needed to come to grips with the truth about my family of origin. She told me there were angelic beings like this, who did not live full human lives. The task, she said, was their true purpose. For want of any other way to apprehend the experience, I chose to believe her. It was the only way to put the event to rest.

CHAPTER 6

THE FATE OF PSYCHOLYTIC
THERAPY IN EUROPE

I have come to accept that the gap between myself and what I perceive as the rest of the world is an integral component of my being, like a supplementary, invisible body part, both omnipresent and formless. It moves and shape-shifts. Once or twice, it has engulfed me entirely, as it did in 2005, when my sister Andrea died. That was the same year I divorced and my house was sold.

A few years on, I managed to find footing again, spanning the chasm with one foot placed over here, the other foot over there, where I imagine the rest of humanity lives. Then, in 2009, I was diagnosed with breast cancer. No job, an economic meltdown, and no health insurance. I was depressed and anxious and horrified at where my health and the state of my career had brought me. I considered suicide. Then, in 2012, came my psilocybin treatment at Johns Hopkins, which unspooled a slim, life-reviving thread in my direction. I twined it in my fingers and held on. I made changes; I moved from England to France, where I could afford to buy a house.

Then came the COVID-19 pandemic. My supposed-to-be-temporary stay in Paris at an apartment belonging to a very old California friend following the sale of my house turned into a year during which I was imprisoned along with my two dogs in a concrete-and-limestone *quartier* near Place de Clichy, where, among other things, men defecated on the sidewalks and loitered drunk and howling half the night on stoops of buildings. I was mugged not once but twice here, the most recent occurrence on the afternoon before Christmas. Fortunately, I was carrying pepper spray. Then, life became really unlivable. Lockdown number three, a comedy *à la Marat/Sade* in which French politicians gamed the population in an endless round of Russian roulette, pitting mortality rates against intensive-care bed counts. After weeks of increasing demoralization, I saw the yawning gap open itself widely in front of me and I toppled in. My working "other," the skilled, well-tooled mechanical bird version of myself, continued to plow ahead. What is that silly saying? Fake it till you make it? I had been unmade. I was not "as if" anything, other than dead.

Life became a series of endless Zoom meetings, human contact reduced to digital interactions. Nothing was personal. People on the street were by turns rude, drunk, or in the midst of committing crimes. I began to feel the way I had felt when I was living in England. I began to wish I were dead.

One day, at an online conference, I heard Dr. Friederike Meckel speak about dosing and combining psychedelic drugs as part of a therapeutic process. She was the rare woman who was versed in psychedelic medicine in what has become a man's world.

Dr. Meckel is best known for her work as a psycholytic therapist, a psychotherapeutic approach augmented through the use of a variety of psychedelic substances, including MDMA, LSD, ayahuasca, and 2C-B, a psychedelic in the phenethylamine family.

First developed by Dr. Hanscarl Leuner in Germany, the practice was initiated in 1960 at the First European Symposium on Psychotherapy under LSD-25 at Göttingen University.

Dr. Meckel has studied and worked extensively. She has practiced family systems therapy, family constellation therapy, hypnotherapy, neurolinguistic programming, and Holotropic Breathwork, a technique developed by Dr. Stanislav Grof and Christina Grof. The Grofs worked with LSD-assisted psychotherapy during the 1960s and 1970s. They developed the Holotropic Breathwork technique when psychedelics were no longer available. Dr. Meckel discovered psychotherapy with substances following her own breakdown in her forties.

The day after we spoke, she texted me. "Dear. How are you? Are you okay?"

I decided I could talk to her. I told her I wasn't okay. I could no longer stand the isolation and demoralization of being in Paris. She invited me to visit her and her husband at their home in Zurich. After much paperwork, and a COVID-19 vaccine obtained by the grace of an acquaintance who headed the infectious diseases vaccination clinic at a Paris hospital, I traveled to Zurich, a four-hour train ride from Paris. For me, accepting an invitation like this was new, different, and entirely out of character.

WHO IS FRIEDERIKE MECKEL?

Dr. Meckel is probably best known for an incident she'd like to forget: the day in 2009 when she was arrested for running psycholytic therapy sessions long after the ban on psychedelic medicine had gone into effect in Switzerland.

Dr. Meckel trained as a medical doctor in Germany and started her career working as a specialist in industrial medicine. She spent many years as the on-site medical doctor in a factory, where she dealt with workplace health and safety issues. She was married and had three children. Then, between the work—she was working day and night shifts—and the children, she fell into something she described as a "life crisis."

"I didn't know what a burnout was until I had one," she said. "Then, on top of all this work, I fell in love with another man."

She got into trouble, she said, because the guy rejected her. She learned he was using her to extract himself from his own marriage, not because of who she was, or because he loved her. She was undone emotionally.

At the time, she was working in the plant as a specialist in workers' health. She had a woman client who had some emotional problems. Dr. Meckel referred her to a former professor of hers, a gynecologist who had started experimenting with breathwork. The woman came back transformed.

"I thought, if she can go there in a crisis, I can go there too," said Dr. Meckel.

Dr. Meckel made an appointment. The doctor put her in a room, placed headphones over her ears, and instructed her in the basics of breathwork.

Dr. Meckel started breathing. Then, she cried for hours. She returned every week for months. She was guided through interior journeys of "deserts, hot deserts, cold deserts, stony deserts," she said.

When Dr. Grof traveled to Munich to lead a workshop in the technique, she attended. There, she came to understand for the first time the far-reaching possibilities of the altered mental state—evoked by controlled breathing at that time—as a means of accessing interior emotional and psychological spaces. Dr. Meckel enrolled in a training course with Dr. Grof in the United States. During the training, Dr. Grof began speaking about psychedelics. She had no idea what he was talking about.

Back at home, the same doctor who had introduced her to breathwork told her about a place where people could meet clandestinely and take psychedelic drugs.

"Sixty people met in an old coal-mine church in the middle of Germany, secretly," she said. Then they were given a pill to swallow. They lay on the floor with headphones all connected to each other. That was in 1989. The drug they'd been given was MDMA.

"I immediately went into a similar state like Holotropic Breathwork but much, much deeper. It lasted eight hours, one dose of MDMA," she said. She recognized immediately that MDMA could be used therapeutically.

The chemical compound, 3,4-methylenedioxymethamphet-amine—MDMA—was originally developed as an intermediate chemical involved in the production of a styptic (a compound that stops bleeding), hydrastinine. It is a phenylisopropylamine derived from safrole, an aromatic oil found in sassafras, nutmeg, and other plants. The drug manufacturer Merck patented MDMA in 1912. Human investigations did not begin until the 1950s, when the US Army began animal experiments, possibly to explore developing the compound for use as a drug for enhanced interrogation.

The chemist Alexander Shulgin, who for many years ran a psychopharmacology experimentation lab in his Lafayette, California, garden shed, gave MDMA he had formulated to a psychotherapist friend, Leo Zeff, in Oakland, California. In the 1970s, Zeff became the first therapist to use it as a psychotherapeutic adjunct.

In 1978, Dr. Shulgin and chemist and pharmacologist David E. Nichols published a report on the drug's psychoactive effect in humans. They described MDMA as inducing "an easily controlled altered state of consciousness with emotional and sensual overtones. It can be compared in its effects to marijuana, to psilocybin devoid of the hallucinatory component."[1]

MDMA is an empathogen—a drug that produces feelings of emotional communion, oneness, and openness. Interpersonal boundaries can blur. Neurochemically, the drug works by causing a decrease in activity in the amygdala—the brain structure associated with memory formation and emotional response—and an increase in activity in the prefrontal cortex—the brain region where cognitive functions are processed, including ethical judgments. It also produces a marked increase in levels of the neurohormone oxytocin, the so-called love hormone, which plays a role in social bonding.

MDMA is also an "entactogen," or a drug that touches from within. MDMA unsticks PTSD sufferers from rigid patterns of emotional reaction brought about by fear. Drugs like MDMA are catalysts, allowing patients to process changes in their own feelings.

Although it would take her some time to identify it, Dr. Meckel later came to understand her own anguish was trauma-related, as the result of both the generational trauma of the war and the sudden death of her father. Although he'd survived the war itself, he was murdered a few years afterward, when she was a young child.

After she'd attended several sessions at the church, someone betrayed the group, and it was disbanded.

At that time, Switzerland was enjoying a brief stay from the ban on therapy with psychedelics. Between 1988 and 1993, the country relaxed its draconian, anti-psychedelic drug laws. Seven psychiatrists were given permission to use the substances in therapy. All seven were members of the Swiss Medical Society for Psycholytic Therapy. One of them offered training sessions in which Dr. Meckel took part.

Psycholytic therapy involves psychedelic-assisted psychotherapy with repeated low-to-moderate drug doses—as opposed to traditional "psychedelic" psychotherapy, which involves a single or infrequent use of a high dose of the drug followed by integration sessions.

Still living in Germany, Dr. Meckel decided then to complete training in psychotherapy. In the meantime, she'd met the man who would become her second husband, a Swiss lawyer, Konrad Fischer. He had come to her first as a counseling patient, a fact that I initially dismissed as unimportant but later found troubling. I learned the counseling detail was pivotal to what transpired during the time I was their guest.

She realized that if he didn't understand the work she was becoming involved in, the relationship wouldn't work. Together, they undertook three years of training in Switzerland.

She studied the uses of MDMA and LSD, psilocybin and 2C-B (4-Bromo-2,5-dimethoxyphenethylamine). She learned how to combine two or three drugs as part of extended drug therapy sessions. Once she completed the training, she moved permanently to Switzerland, where she discovered that the medical bureaucracy would not accept her German medical qualifications.

In 1997, Dr. Meckel and another woman set up a psychotherapeutic and Holotropic Breathwork practice. She continued to work with private clients on the side, sometimes incorporating psychedelics as adjuncts to the therapy. Since she didn't have a regular job, she had time to educate herself. She traveled throughout Europe and the United States taking courses in various psychotherapeutic training modalities in order to enrich herself and her practice.

Dr. Meckel carried out her clinical psychedelic work entirely underground. At one point, after she'd supervised a Holotropic Breathwork workshop at a German monastery, the monastery's head took her aside. He asked if she could spend some time with a few of the meditation students who had, he said, "gotten stuck." She did a few MDMA sessions with them, and they became unstuck. For Friederike, though, the real therapeutic elixir wasn't with individuals in therapy but with groups.

"The group is something very special," she said. In the context of a group psychedelic session, they were "communicating [as if] the group was the world." It was very effective. "People helped each other, we would have talks where they would give feedback, or they did constellation work, where someone would be the mother of someone else, they would have a real relationship so these issues could be dealt with during the session."

She began holding regular group meetings, all clandestine, all word of mouth. She'd work with groups of sixteen or more, using MDMA, LSD, and 2C-B. She avoided psilocybin.

"Mushrooms," she said, "as well as ayahuasca, are teachers. Teacher plants are distinct from the purely chemical substances LSD and MDMA." She continued, "Psilocybin is a teacher plant.

It wants to talk to you. I didn't want to talk," she said. "You have a relationship with the substance you take. It's not just you're taking it. You truly have to enter a relationship. You're not just taking a substance and having it work for you," she said.

"With a normal psychoactive substance [the chemical compounds LSD or MDMA] you can say, 'I ask myself' so you are both subject and object. On a teacher plant, you don't ask yourself, you ask the plant. Then you wait for the answer. The answer is so different from what one answers to oneself. Especially with ayahuasca. It gives you answers you would have never thought of."

On occasion, said Dr. Meckel, she would give psilocybin mushrooms to patients, but only if they were having individual experiences. She couldn't allow them to talk to one another, unless they were on the descent stage—in other words, returning to the shared, consensual reality.

"Mushrooms can be very funny. Then a group starts laughing. It's, like, contagious and you cannot stop them." Ayahuasca, by contrast, she said, is not that funny. "Ayahuasca can get angry," she said. "I once asked the ayahuasca a question twice. She took me and threw me on the floor—*whap*—like a wet cloth. 'You asked me that question yesterday.' So these sessions I did for myself in Brazil. For me, ayahuasca is the deepest substance there is for the very difficult questions," she said.

Using their large house in Zurich, Dr. Meckel and her husband developed an ongoing underground practice in the basement—a huge room with lots of sunlight. The groups met on weekends. She'd spend days cooking, baking, and preparing. Group members arrived on Friday evening. They'd spend Friday, Saturday, and Sunday together. Fridays were to prepare participants for their journey, Saturdays they'd journey, and Sundays were daylong integration sessions.

"Then," she said, "the big thing happened."

In 2009, Dr. Meckel and her husband were arrested. A former client, who had been married to one of Dr. Meckel's long-term therapy clients, decided the breakup of her marriage was Dr. Meckel's doing. She'd reported the psycholytic therapy groups taking place at Dr. Meckel's house to the police. They'd been doing covert surveillance for over a year.

The story actually started a few years before, in 2006, when the woman who ultimately betrayed them had sought Dr. Meckel's professional help in conventional one-on-one talking therapy. She complained bitterly about her husband and was considering divorce. She spent several sessions talking about the difficulties in the marriage. Dr. Meckel offered to speak to the husband as well. She herself didn't do couples counseling but was willing to see the husband alone. He was—and still is—a prominent surgeon in Zurich. He arrived and told her, simply, he was dying. The marriage was a problem, but what was really bothering him, it emerged, was something from childhood. After a few sessions, she invited him to a single psychedelic session with MDMA. It went well, and she invited him to attend one of her weekend group sessions. Since she was no longer seeing the wife, Dr. Meckel recommended a couples' counselor. The couple went to see the counselor together only once. After a few weekend psycholytic group sessions, the husband decided it might help if his wife, Dr. Meckel's original client, attended the groups too.

"It was stupid not to involve the wife again," said Dr. Meckel, when I spoke with her the first time. "Whatever I did would have been wrong. If she came, it was wrong; if I excluded her, it was wrong."

The wife and husband attended several weekend psycholytic sessions together. At the time, she praised Dr. Meckel for their positive experiences using MDMA and LSD.

All the while, Dr. Meckel continued to see the husband individually to address his problems and the issues around his childhood, which were very deep. He did not let on to Dr. Meckel what was actually going on with the marriage.

More than a year passed, and the couple went off to Christmas at a relative's house. Shortly thereafter, the couple had a showdown.

The wife, it emerged, had been opening the husband's private correspondence and had already spoken with an attorney. They separated and the husband moved out. Because he had no place to stay, Dr. Meckel and her husband offered him lodging while he was in a state of transition.

"It was," she recognized, "a big mistake."

He eventually found an apartment of his own, and divorce proceedings got underway. Soon, Dr. Meckel learned the wife was blaming Dr. Meckel for her husband's decision to end the marriage.

Following her husband's departure, she reported Dr. Meckel to the police, embroidering her story to include numerous falsehoods, according to Dr. Meckel. She'd told the police that Dr. Meckel and her husband had used MDMA to "brainwash" her husband and turn him against her. She denied any positive aspects of the sessions she'd had. It was at this time the police put Dr. Meckel's house under surveillance and tapped her telephone and email, searching for evidence of drug dealing.[2]

"Then comes the story no one believes," said Dr. Meckel when I spoke with her.

On Easter 2008, she invited her former patient and his brother to her house for dinner. Dr. Meckel's daughter, her husband, and her three children, who were visiting from Germany, were also there. They all had Easter dinner together, and her daughter and the former patient fell in love. Her daughter revealed the romance to Dr. Meckel when they attended a seminar together later that year. Her daughter left her own husband in Germany in late 2008 and moved to Switzerland with her three children. In 2009, she gave birth to her fourth child, a boy, Dr. Meckel's eighth grandchild.

Four weeks after the grandson was born, Dr. Meckel and her husband were arrested.

In October 2009, the police raided the home and found four tablets and two capsules of MDMA and four tabs of blotter LSD. They seized the couple's computers. They took Dr. Meckel and her husband into custody and sent them to separate prisons. They were interrogated. But, try as they might, the police could find no evidence to suggest they were dealing drugs.

Dr. Meckel was in prison for thirteen days. For five days, she was alone. Then she was moved to another facility where she had a roommate.

"I enjoyed prison life," she said. "In prison, you are sort of protected."

I didn't really understand what she meant until later on. Then I learned about what the press was doing with her story.

On November 11, Dr. Meckel was called in front of the prosecutor, who told her she could go "home and wait for your trial." Then, said Dr. Meckel, "the hard times started."

In January 2010, when newspapers were in their customary postholiday news vacuum, they began running scathing articles. The reporting was abusive, said Dr. Meckel, creating fake narratives in true tabloid style. Her self-esteem was ruined. One journal published a caricature of her as a witch mixing poisons together.

In July 2010, her case went to trial.

Dr. Meckel and her husband were charged with dealing drugs, making a profit from dealing illegal substances, and endangering society. The prosecutor argued that LSD was an intrinsically dangerous drug. The prosecutor did not, however, suggest MDMA was a dangerous drug. Under Swiss law, MDMA is not considered toxic.

A number of influential psycholytic therapists and neuroscientists (Ede Frecska, Peter Gasser, Stanislav Grof, David Nichols, Rick Strassman, and Michael Winkelman) testified on behalf of Dr. Meckel and her husband. LSD, they said, is neither a dangerous drug nor does it have significant physical or psychological adverse effects when given in a controlled, clinical setting. This group of luminaries found that the assertion that the couple were endangering society with their use of LSD was baseless. Set and setting, both necessary to effective therapeutic use of psychedelic drugs, had been adhered to throughout their psycholytic therapy practice. Furthermore, the project was neither profitable nor was it intrinsically about drug dealing for recreational or hedonistic use. Rather, the substances were being used with great care and attention in the context of a therapeutic setting.

Dr. Meckel submitted supportive literature from Albert Hofmann, the Swiss chemist who first synthesized LSD, and Dr. Torsten Passie, a leading expert in psycholytic psychotherapy.

At one point, Dr. Meckel addressed the judge directly. "For me psychedelics like MDMA and LSD are not drugs. They are psycho-integrative substances that have been used for thousands of years. [It] is not like getting drunk. The clients are in a clear state of elevated consciousness in which they can carry out psychotherapeutic work."[3]

Ultimately, Dr. Meckel was found guilty of possession of a small amount of LSD. The sentences were relatively lenient.

Dr. Meckel's husband was fined 10,000 Swiss francs—about $11,000—and was put on a two-year probation. Dr. Meckel was fined 2,000 Swiss francs—about $2,200—and given a sixteen-month suspended sentence and probation of two years.

A Psycholytic Therapy Day

I arrived at the home of Dr. Meckel—Friederike, as she preferred to be called—on April 1, the same day when, a dozen years before, I had received my breast cancer diagnosis. The next day was Good Friday, Easter weekend.

Although I knew that Friederike no longer practiced psycholytic therapy officially, I'd decided in advance that if I were offered a session, I would accept it. I was not going to ask.

Friederike met me at the station. She's diminutive, maybe five feet tall. Her hair was cut close to her head. She wore round glasses, which accentuated her round face. She had a quickness, a lightness to her movements. She reminded me of an owl, an impression underscored by the many owl images and sculptures that decorated her house. Friederike and I rode the street-car to her house, not far from the center of Zurich. Konrad, her husband, and their enormous Weimaraner, Yago, greeted me. The house had three stories as well as a full basement. There was a broad, walled garden with a magnolia tree, apple trees, flower beds, and a kitchen garden to one side. Flowers were just beginning to bloom. Both Konrad, who was an attorney, and Friederike had in-home offices. Since the arrest, Konrad had given up his law license, although he continued an arbitration practice.

When she is not seeing clients, Friederike spends a lot of time cooking and baking for her extended family. The day I arrived, she was baking *Zopf*, a white loaf shaped into a braid, and a German specialty, a dark, full-grain bread. Her kitchen was equipped with every possible high-tech tool. When her group psycholytic therapy practice was active, she'd do all the cooking for the groups who came to stay for the weekend therapy sessions.

That evening, her daughter stopped by and a discussion ensued about the weekend. As it turned out, her family—daughter, son-in-law, and Konrad—had an annual Easter tradition, a group psycholytic therapy session, in partial commemoration of the sequence of events that had brought her daughter and son-in-law together in the first place. It was agreed I'd join them for a session on Saturday morning.

Friederike's group therapy room occupied about a third of her huge basement. It was light and airy, despite being partly underground. She saw clients for therapy, family systems, family constellation therapy, hypnotherapy, and, were it not for COVID-19, Holotropic Breathwork in smaller adjoining rooms.

Early Saturday morning, I watched Friederike's son-in-law weigh 120 milligrams of crystalline MDMA on a precision laboratory scale. He was a world-class hand surgeon. He was never careless. I'd never seen MDMA before. The MDMA photos on the Web invariably depicted colored pressed-powder tablets stamped with logos of smiley faces or elephants. Friederike said she'd kept the MDMA for over twenty years. Stored in airtight containers, crystalline MDMA kept much better than the powdered version because it neither absorbs water nor contains any organic molecules, which can decompose.

When her house was raided in 2009, the police impounded the drugs they found, a few blotter squares of LSD and a few tabs of MDMA. Where, then, did the twenty-odd-year-old MDMA crystals come from?

"I'd stored it in a five-kilo box of washing powder," she said. "They didn't look in there."

At about ten in the morning, we all went into the session room. Konrad carried downstairs a tray laden with doses, each in a shot glass. Friederike and her son-in-law were drinking 2C-B, a psychedelic in the phenethylamine family; Konrad, Friederike's daughter, and I were taking MDMA. Like shamans in ayahuasca or peyote ceremonies, Friederike took some of the substance with the participants. She said it affected her differently. She didn't have the intensity of feeling or disassociation because she was occupied with the participants in the session.

Friederike had covered the foam pads in the room with coverlets. Mine was a cashmere shawl with a silk back, a gift from Konrad when they first met years prior. Friederike's daughter and son-in-law were placed on one side of the room under the ground-level window, beside each other, Konrad opposite them. Friederike's pad was arranged against the adjacent wall, and mine was placed beside hers. She said she wanted me to be close by because I'd never been through this experience before. Konrad passed out the tray, pointing to the glass intended for me.

I swallowed my MDMA. The liquid was bitter, reminiscent of the taste of penicillin tablets from my childhood when, resisting taking them and unable to swallow them whole, I'd crunched them instead.

Friederike asked me about my expectations.

I have some natural gifts I'm proud of, but the one I've come to cherish more and more over the past decade is the ability to go into a situation without expectations.

I really did not have any preconceived notions about what would happen, or what should happen, or what might happen that day. I was entirely in the present.

Friederike started up the music and instructed me to lie down. The music was varied: tribal and traditional music, gongs, an instrument plucked like a harp. After some time had passed, she leaned over and whispered in my ear. She said I should be feeling the effects of the drug. She asked how I was. I said I felt as though nothing was happening. Time did not seem to be passing.

She said, "You should be arriving at a sensation, a plateau now." Then she turned the music off, and everyone sat up.

Friederike asked how everyone was and if they had anything they wanted to address. Both her daughter and son-in-law had specific work they wanted to do. For the daughter, who had been having some physical issues, Friederike decided a reenactment of her daughter's birth would help. The daughter's birth had been a terrible experience for both involved: She was breech (turned the wrong way around) as well as placenta previa, where the placenta covers the birth canal and the baby can't get out. She had almost died of oxygen deprivation; Friederike had almost died from blood loss. Her daughter was ultimately delivered by cesarean section. Konrad and the son-in-law then assisted in the reenacted birth scene.

Next Friederike went to her son-in-law, who was having difficulty with someone who worked for him: a surgeon who had botched a surgery. His difficulty expressing his dismay, he felt, stemmed from his childhood relationship with his brothers. Konrad and Friederike's daughter enacted a scenario with the brothers.

Then Friederike asked me how I felt about what I was seeing. I replied I was witnessing an experience among people that was authentic and deeply felt. I was learning something about those

involved and about myself and how I responded to an emotionally meaningful experience. She wanted to know if what I was
seeing was something that would be done in the United States,
if someone like Charlie Grob had done such a thing. I'd never
heard anything about this kind of therapy in the States. I said I
had no idea.

"Okay," she said. "Now it's your turn." She asked me how I felt.
Did I notice anything? I felt lightheaded, muzzy, as though my
being had been swathed in yards of cotton batting. My lower torso
from navel downward was now weighted with fifty pounds of lead.

I tried to speak. My lips would not move—rather they were
moving, but words failed me. I finally managed to say:

"I'm having trouble speaking."

"But how do you feel?" said Friederike.

I tried to characterize the feeling in my abdomen but could
only come out with "heavy."

She asked me to associate the heaviness with the name of a
feeling. Was it sadness?

"It's just heavy," I said. "As though I can't move."

Friederike's son-in-law from his mat beside his wife said, "You
know you can say anything in here, it's a safe space, no one judges."

I told him as best I could it wasn't about feeling safe. I couldn't
form words.

Friederike moved close to me. She looked at me squarely, her
eyes near mine, unflinchingly, trying to ascertain what I felt.

"Is it fear?" she asked. "Numbness? Sadness? Pain?"

I knew it wasn't pain. Maybe sadness.

"Okay," said Friederike. "Not fear. I think it's numbness and
sadness."

Even at the time, when my mouth and throat refused to work,
I found it ludicrous I could not form sentences.

I live and die by narrative. From the time I was very young,
narrative has been my single tool for making sense of a world
that made no sense. I had, then, the sudden revelation that I use

narrative as a way of avoiding pure feeling. If I could create a story, I could move out of the realm of pain. Transferring the feelings to the world of language made it possible for me to transform overwhelming feelings, bit by tiny bit, into something less deadly. Narrative for me over the decades had been an exercise in defanging. A way to make feelings safe.

Her daughter then asked if she could come over, if she could touch me. I said yes. She put her hand on my lower abdomen and asked me to tell her where the heaviness was. Was it below my pubic bone? I shook my head. No, not genital. She moved her hand up my belly till it was resting below my ribs, above my hips. It was there.

"It's here," she said. "It's about trust. It's about your mother."

Friederike, who knew something about me from my writing, said, "We're going to work on trust." If the heaviness was preverbal and I couldn't identify it, it had to be about my mother.

I protested. I'd spent a decade in therapy, in endless conversation about family issues, coming to terms with the abuse, my ostracism at the hands of the extended family, my parents' determination that I should glorify and gratify their noxious, fabricated world or, if I insisted on being myself, that I fail or die in the attempt. Despite the dedication of Chet—the therapist I saw in my thirties—the changes that did come about did so through means other than speaking, experiences that forced me to remain entirely present and in touch with my physical body. I'd learned by the time I was in my thirties to seek out situations that kept me within the realm of the immediate, where I could not disassociate. These usually involved extreme physical exercise: riding horses, the Model Mugging workshop, running for miles. I simply did not want to revisit my mother in therapy again.

"No matter," said Friederike. "We start somewhere, it's a good place to start. Very simple. We'll see about trust."

She asked me to make statements about my mother, about the beatings that had occurred largely at night during my childhood.

The violence was covert, hidden. Even after I'd aged out of the "she won't dare tell" phase, she found other, crueler ways to torture me that few outsiders ever observed. The family system was designed that way. The abuser was always protected. I was cut off from any part of the world that might have protected me from them.

Friederike sat in front of me and looked intently into my face. She asked me to make "I" statements, to demand that my mother not beat me. She wanted me to do it without losing the present, the frame of reference of the session room, of the here and now.

"Please don't beat me," I said. Evidently, my delivery was rote and not convincing.

"No. That's not working. You're not staying here. Look at me. Say, 'I am Erica. I am here.'"

I said, "I am Erica."

"And I am Friederike. Who am I?"

"You? You're Friederike."

"Again," she said. "Who am I?"

"Friederike."

"And who are you?"

"Erica."

"Say it, the whole thing: 'I am Erica.'"

"I am Erica," I said.

She knew when I was speaking with an overlay of dispassion or when I was absenting myself emotionally—a habit with trauma survivors that is so automatic we often can't prevent ourselves from doing it.

Emotional work does not take place in the cerebral cortex, where language originates. Emotional work requires a person to remain in an integrated state with free-flowing access to the limbic system, a mid-brain structure that retains a record of memories around behaviors that produced agreeable and disagreeable experiences during developmental stages.[4]

Development of this brain level occurs in the first years of life. Unlike the so-called lizard brain—the autonomic nervous system, which includes functions such as heart rate, pupil dilation, sexual arousal, and the fight-or-flight instinct, which forms in the very earliest stages of development and is essentially unchangeable—the midbrain encapsulates the core of personality. Emotions such as joy, fear, contempt, disgust, and curiosity develop here. These emotions tend to be fixed by adulthood and can change in adolescence and in adulthood only through intense or long-lasting emotional experiences. This, then, is how MDMA works: It causes the pathway between the limbic, emotion-forming brain and the upper language-speaking, rational-thought-forming cognitive part of the brain to open and remain that way for several hours. Or, rather, it prevents that particular hatch from slamming shut. The fear reaction, sparked by recalled trauma, is suppressed for a time.

Days afterward, I realized this was probably why I was having such difficulty speaking during the session. With the aid of MDMA, the conscious, judgmental, language-forming part of my mind had been superseded, temporarily, by the emotional. I had no choice but to be present with my feelings. Evidently, for me, on that day, this could occur only by way of the banishment of words.

Friederike asked me if I trusted her.

I said I did. I added, with difficulty, that having gotten on a train to come stay with people I didn't know was out of character for me. I had trusted Friederike from the first time I spoke with her. The experience, the timing especially, became even more uncanny in hindsight, when, three weeks later, I learned that my father had finally died, at the age of ninety-seven, on April 1, the same day I'd arrived in Zurich at Friederike and Konrad's. I'm convinced he'd spent the weeks before his death cursing my very life. I wasn't supposed to have outlived him. It was clear to me from the time I was very young that, as far as he and my mother were concerned, I was supposed to have died. But I left. The wrong child died: my younger sister, Andrea.

Friederike asked her daughter to come over and play the role of my mother. She sat on her knees in front of me.

"Can you speak to her?" asked Friederike. "She's your mother, you are Erica."

I averted my gaze and looked over her shoulder. Friederike asked me to look at her daughter, who was a doctor and has one of the kindest faces I've ever seen. I knew she'd been through numerous sessions with Friederike. I had every confidence she knew what she was doing in the session.

With difficulty—my mouth simply did not want to open—I said, "If she's my mother, I have nothing to say to her. I don't trust her."

"Okay," said Friederike. "You don't trust her." She leaned in front of her daughter and placed her face directly in front of mine.

"Who am I?" she said.

"Friederike."

She said, "What do you feel when you look at Friederike?"

"I feel fine."

"Do you trust Friederike?"

"Yes."

"Okay."

"I wouldn't have come here had I not trusted you. I never do this kind of thing. This is something I don't do."

She said, "Okay. Now, look at her. She's your mother."

It was as though Friederike could read my interior.

"What would you like to say to your mother?"

"Nothing."

"Your mother beat you. Tell her not to beat you."

"What do I say?"

"You say, 'Mommy, don't beat me.'"

I said, "Mommy, don't beat me." Her daughter didn't find it convincing.

"No, it's not there. You're above it. You're not there," she said. She was as keyed into vocal intonation and subtext as was Friederike. I was having a terrible time addressing her daughter as my mother. I couldn't do it. She sat on her knees in front of me, her gaze unbending.

Then Friederike moved closer to me and placed her face in front of mine, obscuring my view of her daughter. She asked me to look at her and not look away.

She repeated, "I'm Friederike. Who are you?"

"I am Erica," I said.

"Who am I?"

"You are Friederike."

"And you are?"

"I am Erica."

"Okay," she said. Then with her face very close to mine, so I could almost feel her breath, she asked, "What do you see here? Do you see an emotion? Can you describe it?"

I saw then someone who actually cared about my well-being. Affection, concern, fellow-feeling. It was an astonishing moment.

She said, "Can you see what I am feeling right now? Do you recognize it?"

I described her look.

She said, "You're able to see this when it's in front of you. That's already good. Some can't recognize affection when they see it."

She moved her head away and said, "Now, you talk to her, she's your mother. Tell her how you feel. Tell your mother to stop beating you."

She watched me fixedly.

I said, "Please don't beat me."

Friederike's daughter said, "No, it's not there. Above, below. Not there."

Friederike said, "Can you trust her?"

I said, "Not if she's my mother. I can trust you, but not my mother. I know who my mother is."

"What do you want to do to your mother?"

"Nothing," I said. "I don't feel anything, other than I don't trust her."

It was an absence. Nothing else.

"What would you like to do to her?"

"If you're asking if I want to hit her or punch her, the answer is no. I can't hurt anyone. That isn't who I am."

Friederike looked at me intently. "Who are you?"

"I am Erica."

"And who am I?"

"You are Friederike."

"And you trust me."

"Yes. I trust you. I don't trust her."

"Tell her how you feel."

Eventually, I was able to tell her how I felt.

"I don't trust you," I said. "I wanted you to stop beating me. I asked you to stop beating me."

The conversation proceeded a bit from there. One of the insights Friederike's daughter provided was the essential fact of my being small and helpless, and my mother was a grown-up and could do what she wanted. From that emerged the insight that my mother had somehow expected me to take care of her, and that part of the beating was her frustration. No one was looking after her, evidently, and somehow the responsibility had fallen to me. Helplessness engulfed me. I had an insight then about a passivity that has overwhelmed me, at times, in situations where I should have known how to act. A small child. Three years old. She asked me to tell her daughter how little I was, how I was a child and helpless.

"Say it to her. 'I am only little.'"

Her daughter repeated, "Say it to me. 'I am only little. You are big. I can't take care of you.'"

I repeated the words. She nodded. "That was good. You were there."

Then she said, "But what about the good times? Can you remember the good times? There must have been some good times."

I looked at Friederike.

"Answer her, she's your mother," said Friederike.

"There are none."

"None?" said Friederike's daughter.

"No."

Friederike was looking at me intently. Her daughter looked at me.

"I don't know what to say," I said. "That's how it is."

"If that's how it is, that's how it is," said Friederike.

I looked at her daughter and saw her, sitting in front of me on her knees. She was the mother of four children ranging in age from eleven to early twenties. I recognized how profoundly difficult it must have been for her to envision how any real mother could have behaved the way mine did. I felt bad for her.

"I know you, as yourself, have a terrible time seeing how any real mother could behave the way mine did," I said. "I am aware how difficult it must be to see it. I know you are a good mother; I would like to recall a good moment, but there were none. She was always drunk or wanted me to take care of her, or beating me, or setting the children against one another. I know in my heart you aren't that way. I would have loved to have you as a mother. Any child who has you as a mother is blessed."

"Okay," interjected Friederike. "She is fine with herself. Now tell me if there is something you can remember in which you felt joy. Anything. Any moment in childhood. Your mother doesn't have to be part of it."

I remembered an incident with my sister Andrea, when she and I were small. We were playing marbles in the waiting room of my father's office. It must have been winter and snowing; otherwise, we'd have played on the sidewalk outside. I'd formed a circle with a piece of white string, the kind used decades ago to tie packages. We had all the marbles out—two jars' worth—big ones, little ones, cats' eyes, aggies, steelies, all of them. We must have played for a good hour. I recall the unevenness of the rug deflected a few good shots. We permitted each other to rearrange moves when the rug got in the way. I was about seven. Andrea must have been four. My mother was there. She sat on a chair smoking and watched us dispassionately, for once in her life not trying to destroy my experience with one of my siblings. She let us merely be with one another.

I return to that memory frequently now that Andrea is dead. It seems pure, unencumbered, something authentic from a childhood that was anything but. Even now, I recall time I spent with Andrea with a kind of limpid clarity. My memories of my elder sister and brother are darker, muddier, colored with the sadistic presence of my parents, whose first lieutenants they were and have remained. When my brother-in-law Hayes's call came at three in the morning on September 11, 2005, informing me Andrea had died, I responded in a perfectly calm and rational voice, "Andrea is not dead. I just tied her shoes."

Forty-odd years had tesseracted away, and I was there in Massachusetts, tying her little white Stride Rite shoes.

By the time the session ended, it was almost dark. A good five hours had passed.

As the others stood up, I could not rise. I sat there.

"Are you okay?" asked Friederike. "We're going upstairs to have some food."

"I can't stand up."

"Juice," said Friederike.

Konrad had brought down bottles of sparkling cider, sparkling water, and chocolate. MDMA could affect the metabolism, often speeding it up. Evidently, my blood sugar level had plummeted. I drank a bottle of apple cider. After a few minutes, I stood. Friederike's daughter, close by, came over and asked if she could hug me.

"Of course," I said. I understood then the magic of the group psycholytic session: Therapeutic work happens continuously, with the therapist as well as between and among the participants, through the guided interaction.

The following day, and on each subsequent day, Friederike invited me to speak with her about how I felt—integration work. I was still having trouble articulating my feelings.

After a day, she asked me to sit down with her. We sat at a low table set in a bright space just off the kitchen beside the window. It was a beautiful spring day. The window overlooked the kitchen garden, now fallow, and a budding fruit vine espaliered to a growing frame.

A difficult conundrum emerged, as it has several times, about the abuse. I become two people. One of me—the adult—is supposed to have been present during the worst of my abuse and saved the small child—the three- or four-year-old. This has been my Gordian knot since my thirties.

It was compounded in 2005, when I spoke with Andrea before she died. She, too, felt I should have saved her. She felt that I had abandoned her personally when I divorced my family of origin. I tried to point out to her at the time that I could barely save myself. Whether she would admit it or not, we had entirely different experiences of our mother. I did not have the impression she wanted saving. She detested my father and blamed him for the family psychosis. When we were young, I never thought she would have come away with me.

Friederike wanted me to put this particular paradox away. She reached to a shelf under the table and pulled out a container filled with wooden dolls, each a few inches high. She chose one for me, the small child, and one for me, the adult. She set them on the table. She pointed out I'd locked myself in a circle that I had to get out of. The adult me could not have become the adult if the child had not managed to survive. The child managed. She put the child to one side. The adult came about later and was trying to solve the problem for the child. The child had survived.

Friederike picked up the adult doll. "Here you are. Those two are separate. This one"—she put the adult down on the table in front of me—"has to step out of the circle where she is caught."

It is one of the essential truths about survivors of severe childhood abuse that we blame ourselves for what happened to us. We internalize the message that if we were better than we were, the parent would not have had to do what he or she did.

I hadn't really grokked, until the MDMA session, how I had truly felt, on a purely emotional plane as a child—other than those times when I was reduced to a state of dissociated terror while my parents either beat me or carried out acts of emotional gaslighting so extreme they make the sadistic experiments of Henry Alexander Murray at Harvard seem amateur in comparison.

As a child, I found myself thrown down a well—like the days I spent locked in my father's office, separated from my siblings and banished from even the temporary relief offered by the structured anonymity of kindergarten—in a kind of limbo awaiting an unthinkable fate.

As soon as I learned to read, narrative crept in. I developed an overlay of intellectualisation that appears to me to have been borrowed from my future self, if such a thing is possible.

Even now, revisiting my childhood memories is painful.

At the time, I was incapable of recognizing my smallness and vulnerability in the presence of omnipotent adults. I'd never recognized my feelings for what they were: mostly abject terror, knowing I'd soon be annihilated. I feared for myself and for Andrea who, I knew, even as a child, was in some special way vulnerable in the way I was. But I got away. Andrea, for many reasons, could not. She died because of it. The fact both she and I developed cancer—no other member of the family ever did— was entirely predictable in light of current research: We'd both been severely abused as children.[5] I was physically abused by both parents from the age of three; Andrea was sexually abused by an uncle when she was eight.

Glimpsing a tight circle of blue sky from the bottom of that pit, I never once imagined I'd ever get out. There was no one to reach down a hand and pull me out. I could not pull myself out.

My persistent problem with vulnerability stems from this feeling: *If I'm vulnerable, and small, and down a well, who will help me? How can I get out alone?* The fact is, I couldn't get out alone. *No one could.* As I grew up, I learned I needed others to help me.

Although I will never be able to remake the past, over the last three decades or so, I've gained a sense of a path going forward. It relies on my engagement with other people, even the kinds of people I used to fear. When I can locate myself in the reality of a moment in time and space, then I can trust my capacity to respond in the emotional present in a self-affirming and, if need be, self-protective way. I can trust myself to know at a cellular level how to proceed. I will know how to ask for help when I'm down in the well. I recognize the difference between those who want to help me get out and those who will leave me to die there alone.

If the story stopped here, I could say the experience was perfect. I wanted it to be perfect. I did, after a time, feel I had resolved at least one unresolved childhood issue: who should have been doing the rescuing, which, as a four-year-old, I couldn't do. But the story didn't stop here. I stayed at the Fischer/Meckel household a week.

During the session and during the week that followed, some disturbing things happened. At the time, I did what most of those with CPTSD do when a situation overwhelms us: I pretended it didn't matter. A year-plus on from the experience, I remembered why I had stopped lying to myself in adulthood.

Gaslighting oneself is even worse than having it done to you.

—

CHAPTER 7

THE MEANING OF
THE TRANSPERSONAL

✦

I met Charles S. Grob, professor of psychiatry and pediatrics
at Harbor-UCLA Medical Center and the UCLA School of
Medicine, in 2013 in London at a dinner given by Dr. Robin
Carhart-Harris. We were both scheduled to speak at a conference
at Imperial College that Dr. Carhart-Harris had organized taking
place on the following day. Dr. Grob (whom I address as Charlie)
was the first physician in modern times to carry out a clinical
study using psilocybin. He treated twelve advanced-stage cancer
patients suffering from depression and anxiety with two doses of
psilocybin using a protocol he developed, a precursor to the study
in which I took part.[1] I'd completed the psilocybin study at Johns
Hopkins University in 2012 and written a long article published
in *Scientific American Mind* about the science and the experience.[2]

The night before my talk, I met him and one of the conference
hosts, David Nutt, Edmond J. Safra Professor of Neuropsychopharmacology and director of the Centre for Psychedelic Research
in the Division of Psychiatry, at Imperial College London. At that

time, Imperial had yet to get its first psilocybin clinical trial off the ground. Charlie struck me as genial and emotionally present. His persona was less that of a studious academic than of the kind of person whom I might have encountered a long time ago riding fence lines near my former home in California.

I'd never spoken publicly before and I was nervous. I'd prepared note cards because I was sure I wouldn't remember what I wanted to say. My nerves, Charlie assured me, would become less of a problem the more experienced I became.

Charlie's pathway into psychedelic medicine was anything but direct. He did not know he wanted to become a psychedelic researcher until after he dropped out of Oberlin College in the early 1970s and went to work as an assistant at the Dream Research Laboratory at Maimonides Medical Center in Brooklyn.

As the eldest of four children, Charlie was expected to follow in the footsteps of his father, David, a specialist in internal medicine and world-renowned expert in diseases of the neuromuscular junction, particularly myasthenia gravis. Charlie's mother, Elizabeth, was a nurse.

On Long Island, where he had spent his teenage years, Charlie was not exposed to street-drug use. One day, his mother showed him an article in a glossy magazine with a photo of a woman having a bad trip.

"She said, 'Promise me you'll never do this.' I said, 'Are you kidding? That's not me. I have no interest in that stuff,'" said Charlie.

But that was before he started college in 1968, where he learned for himself what psychedelics were about.

Charlie's mother, Elizabeth, was a German Jewish refugee whose family had come to the United States in 1940, mid-war, narrowly escaping through Sweden. He describes her as "one of the most politically radical people I ever met. She'd go on and on about more women in politics. 'If women were in charge, we'd have a healthier world.'"

The story around Charlie's birth was emblematic of his

mother's take-no-prisoners character. When he was born, in 1950, virtually all women in American hospitals were given scopolamine during birth, a deliriant used to induce amnesia. It was better known as "twilight sleep."

Elizabeth, born in Germany, where childbirth was considered a natural event, informed the obstetrician she wasn't going to sleep; she wanted to be awake for the birth. The doctor refused to allow it. Finally, he relented a bit, on the condition she be placed in arm restraints. Charlie was born with his mother's arms shackled to the table.

What happened next nearly cost Elizabeth her ability to have any more children.

"The head obstetrician took me aside to do my Apgar and said to the new obstetrics intern, 'Help expel the placenta,'" he told me. "This was August. The academic year starts in July. The guy did not have much experience. He goes over to my mother, puts one hand on her belly, and with the other takes hold of the cut end of the umbilical cord, and he starts yanking it. My mother was screaming at him to stop, and he was yelling at her to cooperate and to 'bear down.' She knew he's going to rip her uterus. She's in restraints. So she does the only thing she can do—leans forward and, with all her might, she bit him on the arm. That was my introduction to life: My mother biting the Hopkins doc on the arm. He almost saw to it that I had no siblings. But, fortunately, my mother had sharp teeth. He was furious at her. But she did what she had to do and was proud of it."

Charlie's story of his mother made an uncanny impression on me. It had a profound subliminal impact, which became evident while I was in Zurich.

It was at Oberlin College between 1968 and 1970 when Charlie had his first psychedelic experiences. Charlie, like many of his era, was captivated and intrigued by the stories he'd been hearing about psychedelics. He first tried LSD in his dorm. On one occasion in 1969, he took some acid given to him by an acquaintance. Then he witnessed a theft. Naively, he attempted to confront the thief. That encounter didn't go well, and the experience amplified into something he'd prefer not to have undergone: the proverbial bad trip. Shaken, Charlie went to a friend's room to talk about what had happened, only to find himself watching the faces of the friend and the friend's girlfriend morph into the muzzles of wolves.

"I knew I was hallucinating," he said. "I was definitely triggered. It was the opposite of anything like an optimal set and setting." Fortunately, the friend was knowledgeable about psychedelics and was sympathetic. "He was a decent person," said Charlie, "a kind of group leader in the dormitory." They were able to talk the experience through and help him back to earth. He came down. He decided to try LSD a few months later, just to prove to himself he could do it without unraveling, but after that he did not take any psychedelics for the next twenty years.

Charlie read everything he could find at the time about psychedelics. His eventual career choice was catalyzed by his college experiences.

An urban dweller for most of his life, Charlie found psychedelics opened up the world of nature to him. "I had the sudden realization nature is alive," he said. He began taking long walks out in the countryside in Ohio, where Oberlin College was located.

In the middle of his junior year, Charlie developed infectious mononucleosis and went home to recuperate. When he was feeling better, he left to travel in Europe. A year later, he returned to Oberlin. But after a week back, he felt uncomfortable, out of place, as though he no longer fitted in at all. He decided to return to New York and take more time off. For a while, he tutored kids with learning disabilities in a child psychiatry unit at Coney Island Hospital. Concerned about Charlie's evident lack of direction, David suggested Charlie might be interested in some psychiatry research taking place at the hospital where he worked. The researchers had received a grant from the NIMH to study dreams and transpersonal communication during sleep at the Maimonides Dream Laboratory, founded by Dr. Montague Ullman and Dr. Stanley Krippner.

Charlie met with Dr. Ullman, who gave him a job as an assistant running experiments on dream telepathy, an extrasensory technique where a person in the rapid eye movement (REM) stage of sleep taps into identifiable information sent to them by someone located a distance away.

Despite the fact that the reigning scientific paradigm since the Enlightenment had relegated anything that did not fit with the Newtonian-Cartesian paradigm to the realm of hocus-pocus, the US Department of Defense and the NIMH had developed an interest in "remote viewing" during the Cold War.

Remote viewing is an ability innate in certain people who are able to acquire information about spatially and temporally remote geographical targets otherwise inaccessible by any known sensory means.[3]

US intelligence agencies had learned the Soviets were doing research like this.

"So, if they were interested in it, then we were too," said Charlie.

EXPERIMENTS IN THE DREAM LAB

The Dream Lab was set up for two volunteers, one who was asleep during the experiment (the receiver) and one who remained awake (the sender). Charlie's first task was to place electroencephalogram (EEG) leads on the receiver, take them to a sensory-deprivation chamber where there was a bed, connect the leads to a monitor, and wish them good night.

Next, he'd go to the sender, who was waiting in an office at the end of a hall. He showed them six sealed, numbered, large envelopes, each containing a picture. Charlie did not know what particular images the envelopes contained; the secretary had done

the sealing and numbering. He then handed the sender the envelopes and told them to choose one. Then the sender opened the
envelope and looked at the picture. Charlie told them to study
the picture for twenty minutes, make notes about it, and draw
it—whatever it took to really focus on it. Then the sender put the
picture back in the envelope, returned it to Charlie, and went to
sleep on a couch in the office. Back in the lab, Charlie monitored
the EEG feed of the receiver throughout the night.

"I could tell when they went through a dream," said Charlie,
"because it's manifested on the EEG as a REM episode." He'd
placed EEG leads right in the corner of each eye to track eye
movement as the eyes moved during phases of actual dreaming.
Then when the REM phase ended, at the end of the dream, he
would turn on the intercom and call to the subject. When they
awoke, he'd ask what was going through their mind. They'd give a
dream report. He'd tape-record the report, and the subject would
go back to sleep.

In the morning, he'd retrieve the envelopes, open them, shuffle
the pictures, and give them to the receiver with instructions to
arrange them in the order they believed were the most likely to
have been sent. If the receiver's first three choices included the
picture sent by the sender, they were included in a larger study of
four more dream sessions.

During the next phase of the study, the sender viewed four
short films. Two were intended to be boring and uneventful: a
black-and-white travelogue of London; a promotional video adver-
tising 1960s California as a promising place to relocate business.

Then there were two other brief films that were intended
to be emotionally evocative: one was a close-up, colorful, obstetrics teaching film of a live birth, and one was an anthropological
black-and-white film from the 1930s that showed an adolescent
initiation ceremony in New Guinea that included a circumcision.

One night, the subject was a young woman who seemed to
be sort of spacey. Because Charlie had to remain awake to run the

study, he spent the nights reading. On that particular night, he read a coffee-table book by J. B. Priestley called *Man and Time*.

"I was flipping the pages looking at pictures and reading the discussions of the pictures. Then, at one point, there was a picture of a mummy that had been excavated from an archaeological site. An hour later, the subject had a dream she was in a desert, in Egypt. She saw pyramids protruding from the sand, and she's sliding down the pyramids. I thought, 'Holy shit.' Her dream was [a] direct hit to what I'd been reading."

The sender, meanwhile, had viewed the film of the initiation ceremony with the circumcision. Charlie could not recall whether she picked up on the film.

One of the two founders of the Dream Lab, Stanley Krippner, kept in his office a vast library of books and articles about psychedelics, which he invited Charlie to peruse and borrow. Charlie borrowed frequently and read voraciously.

"So, one night, at about three in the morning, I picked up the phone, called my father, woke him up, and told him I wanted to study psychedelics," said Charlie.

His father responded by telling him his career goals were fine with him, except he would have to get his credentials first if he wanted to be taken seriously.

The First Drug Study

By the time Charlie started medical school in 1975, the mood of the country had changed. The 1960s were over. Having an expansive view of things, breaking boundaries, all of that was rapidly being replaced by a much stodgier and close-minded ethos, a retrenchment into conservatism. The Dream Lab shut for lack of funding. And no one was doing psychedelic research anymore. The door to exploration of the transpersonal appeared closed.

"[Psychedelics] had gone from cutting-edge to not even being in the field. They were not even mentioned in discussions of potential new and novel treatments in psychiatry," said Charlie. It was as though the entire field of psychiatry had said "good riddance" to them. The general medical philosophy was going backward. By the end of medical school, Charlie was disenamored with psychiatry.

"There was not sufficient substance in the standard treatment approach," he said. "I didn't get a sense that existing treatments were effective."

Rather than pursue psychiatry, Charlie decided he would continue his medical training in internal medicine, moving first to San Francisco to train at Pacific Medical Center and then to Stanford University School of Medicine to study neurology.

One day, he happened upon Stanislav Grof's first two books in the Stanford Bookstore. He bought them both and devoured them that weekend.

"[They] reminded me why I went to medical school in the first place. It was like there was a glitch, and for several years it seemed like this path would never be possible again, so I figured I'd go into medicine and help people like my father had."

He transferred to a psychiatry residency at Cedars-Sinai Medical Center in Los Angeles. Despite some initial discouragement with the way the field had gone, he found a way to stick with it. Near his hospital was a bookstore called the Bodhi Tree, where there was an entire shelf devoted to psychedelics. He'd browse there several times a week to see if there were any new books in. And, sometimes, there were.

"Lester Grinspoon's book *Psychedelic Drugs Reconsidered* and Stan Grof's book *LSD Psychotherapy: The Healing Potential of Psychedelic Medicine* came out around then," said Charlie. He slipped back into reading everything he could on the topic. "Still, within the mainstream—this was in the early 1980s—it was not a topic for discussion. The schedule of topics at the national meetings in psychiatry never had anything on this. It had completely vanished."

He completed his residency and was under some pressure to join the psychoanalytic institute. That didn't interest him. He'd discovered during his rotations he liked working with kids. As the eldest brother in a family with four kids, he was a natural fit.

He left for Baltimore to do a residency at Johns Hopkins in child psychiatry. Although there was nothing going on there at the time with psychedelics, he threw himself into his new specialty. At Hopkins, Charlie met an old Spring Grove researcher, psychiatrist Francesco DiLeo.

"DiLeo got himself into a lot of trouble around psychedelics," said Charlie. "He was using psychedelics in his private practice. His specialty was the 'nadir' experience. And he did hit bottom with his behavior. . . . I had to pull back. I didn't want to be associated with him."

DiLeo was later sued by a patient for sexually abusing her. DiLeo, who said the woman needed sexual touching to treat her Oedipal complex, eventually lost his license. DiLeo was hardly the lone ranger in this kind of behavior.[4]

It has continued, and in some ways gotten worse, as psychedelics have begun to enter the mainstream.

As far as psychedelic research was concerned at that time, Baltimore was a nonstarter. Charlie began looking for other positions around the country. He was recruited by the University of California, Irvine. He moved, but he still felt disillusioned about the state of psychiatry.

Then he met senior professor Dr. Roger Walsh, who was a leader in the transpersonal field. At lunch one day, Charlie told him he was so disillusioned with psychiatry he was thinking of going back into internal medicine. He told Walsh he wanted to study psychedelics, yet the subject had vanished from the field, there was no clinical research going on anywhere, and the idea now seemed futile.

Walsh differed. He thought there was a possibility the field would open up again, and Charlie was in an excellent position to do pivotal work. Walsh encouraged him to hang in there.

In one of our many conversations, Charlie described his conversation with Walsh.

"You need to get focused," Walsh told him. "How are you going to get permission to develop a study with psychedelics? Start with writing research reviews."

Although there were no clinical trials going on, Charlie and another junior faculty member, Gary Bravo, began looking for published science on psychedelics. They began writing reviews on MDMA research, which, although made illegal in 1985, was still being studied in animals and was widely used as a street drug.

Then Charlie came across a study published in the *Archives of General Psychiatry* in 1989, declaring MDMA to be neurotoxic.

"It was a very poorly done study," said Charlie. "The methodology was flawed, there were problems with the data analysis, and the conclusions were off base. I didn't even think it was worthy of publication."

Charlie, Bravo, and Walsh wrote a letter to the editor of the *Archives*, "Second Thoughts on 3,4-Methylenedioxymethamphetamine (MDMA) Neurotoxicity." The letter, published in 1990, detailed their critiques and declared the research to be fundamentally flawed.[5]

A few weeks after the letter was published, Charlie received a call from Rick Doblin, the founder and executive director of the Multidisciplinary Association for Psychedelic Studies (MAPS). Psychopharmacologist and author Sasha Shulgin had just shown him Charlie's letter in the *Archives*. Doblin was desperate to speak with him.

"I'd never heard of this character," recalled Charlie. "He said he had to speak with me. He was kind of pushy and talked a lot. He said he was going to be in LA and wanted to visit. So, he visited. He told me about MAPS."

Doblin was looking for an MD to become the principal investigator in a study using MDMA to treat cancer patients suffering from depression. It was not exactly what Charlie wanted to do, but it was similar enough.

Charlie wrote up a protocol and sent it to the FDA. In 1992, the FDA approved the Phase 1 study. As with all Phase 1 studies, its primary purpose was to assess the safety of the drug more than its efficacy.

A safety study on MDMA, though not Charlie's first choice, was his toehold into the field. Once things got rolling, he never looked back.

Charlie's first MDMA study—with a group of eighteen healthy adults—began in 1994, just after New Year's. Shortly thereafter, he traveled to Brazil to conduct a bio-medical-psychiatric study on ayahuasca use in the União do Vegetal.[6] Ten years on, in 2004, his groundbreaking study, using psilocybin to treat depression in terminal cancer patients, got underway. It was this event that put psychedelics back on the medical map after an absence of thirty years.

Transpersonal Encounters in the Web of Family

Although I've known Charlie since 2013, it wasn't until more recently that I came to know him better. I'd been speaking with him for a few months over Zoom, when, in March of 2021, I realized I was becoming unmoored. What was occurring was something more than just the malaise and isolation brought about by the COVID-19 lockdown. Something very strange was happening, and I couldn't tell what it was or where it was coming from.

When Charlie and I met over Zoom in March 2021, I could barely speak in full sentences. I was scanning for words as though I was in a migraine backwash with its resulting aphasia. Charlie and I spoke about how and where I might find help. I wanted nothing to do with the French psychiatric establishment, largely because they're acutely psychoanalytical and they favored inpatient placement for treating depression. The politics and not-so-secret pharma alliances of the director of Paris's main mental hospital, Centre Hospitalier Sainte-Anne, had made intravenous ketamine the preferred drug to treat depression. I wanted nothing to do with it.

We talked about my getting paperwork together to travel to the United States, where I'd wanted to be since 2020. If the project were to involve him, he'd have to fill out and sign attestations affirming that the trip was medically necessary. Otherwise, under the martial law in effect in Paris at the time, I could not travel more than a few kilometers from where I was living, in the 18th arrondissement near Montmartre. It was shortly thereafter that Friederike Meckel Fischer invited me to visit her in Zurich. At the time, her invitation felt like a godsend.

The night after I arrived at Friederike's house, I had a dream much like a recurrent dream I had had when I was in my twenties and thirties:

I am in a building, like an abattoir, supine on a stone bier in the middle of a room. I am so tired that I am unable to move. I want to leave, but I can't—or maybe I simply no longer have the will to do anything. I want to die.

In an earlier iteration of this dream, my own mother and other figures, all of them indistinct, are there ostensibly to help me, to give me something so I feel better. My wrists are cut open and transparent tubing is placed in my veins in order, I presume, to supply me with liquid to revive me. That doesn't happen. Instead of feeling revived, I grow weaker and weaker as I watch my own blood seep away.

But that night, in the dream, I didn't just slip back into nothingness. Instead, a woman suddenly appeared beside me. She was shouting, she was yelling, she was saying, "You don't let them do that to you, you don't!"

I thought, *But what am I to do?*

She shouted at the top of her lungs, "*You bite them!*"

I awoke then, coughing, to find my teeth clamped ferociously around a length of sheet I'd twisted between my hands.

Shortly after I returned to Paris, Charlie and I spoke. Before I told him about the dream, I asked him if his mother, Elizabeth, had been in his thoughts more than usual. Had he spoken about her? He said yes, in fact, his daughter had visited the previous week—while I was in Zurich—and they'd been reminiscing. I told him about the person who came to me in a dream: an inch or two taller than I, a bit heavier, short hair, strong features. Yes, he said, that was Elizabeth.

I told him about the dream and about how I was in that state of paralysis I used to experience as a child and teenager, when I'd lost all ability to withstand what was taking place in my parents' household. The paralysis had recurred for years in dreams, starting with my childhood and continuing through my young adulthood. Often, the paralysis took the form of crippling migraines lasting for days. And here was Elizabeth, at this moment, telling me now was the time to get moving and to take charge. To bite them.

He listened. Then he said, "If she visits you again, please tell her I love her."

A week later, on April 17, I received a message from my elder sister informing me of my father's death. He had died on April 1, 2021, the same day I had set out for Switzerland, the same date, twelve years before, I'd received my breast cancer diagnosis.

It was then that I understood what Elizabeth was trying to tell me, and what had been happening to me in March: My father, across years and oceans, was making a desperate attempt to bring me under his thumb before he died.

My experience with Charlie's mother in my dream was not my first transpersonal or emergent experience. Far from it.

My sister Andrea was born when I was three and a half. When she came home from the hospital, a crib was set up for her in my father's office waiting room, across the hall from the kitchen. I visited her as frequently as I could, taking hold of her hand, which would wind its little fingers around my thumb. But she had something wrong with her heart, and only I knew about it. I knew what a heart was, how it lived in the chest and pumped the blood. I knew how a heart was supposed to look: red, round, like a cartoon heart. But hers kept appearing to me as malformed. Where its surface was supposed to be smooth and bright crimson, hers was wrinkly and grayish. I may have tried to tell my mother there was something wrong. I would have been summarily ignored. I became obsessed with her fragility.

Nights I would pray to whatever simulacrum of "God" I could come up with to spare Andrea's life. I bargained with this deity. Could he please give Andrea some more life and take some of my parents'? They were already old. They'd lived their lives and didn't need much more. Perhaps cut a piece of life off the end of theirs and sew it onto Andrea's?

I spent as much time with her as I was allowed. I remember the day she took her first step when she was one, in the dining room, grabbing the lower shelf of the sideboard and hoisting herself to her feet.

When Andrea was five, her heart failed during surgery to remove her adenoids. The surgeon stumbled across a heart valve defect that had gone previously undetected. Even after she was released from the hospital, I worried about her. I never stopped worrying about her. I knew she would die young. Or I would. Or both of us would.

After I cut ties with my family of origin for good and began to gain some confidence about my place in the world, I began to let my guard down. I stopped worrying. I didn't hear anything about her for years, and because my interdiction against family applied uniformly to all of them, she did not have my contact information either, despite the fact I would have liked to be in touch with her. My parents, having no boundaries, would harass any sibling they thought might have my contact information until the information was forked over.

Then one day, in my forties, I learned she was dying. The premonition from decades before landed like a neutron bomb at my feet.

At the time I received my elder sister's email in 2021, I had not seen my father in over thirty years. I had had only one communication with him—if you could call it that—in more than three decades, in 2016. That final interchange consisted of my father's surprise invasion of my California lawyer's office. He would have been ninety-two.

According to my attorney, he burst into his office unannounced one morning demanding my signature on a notarized document stating I wouldn't go after his estate when he died. My query about my mother's will—if there was one—was what provoked him, evidently. I had not been notified of her death but rather learned of it accidentally. My mother had died of Lewy body dementia in 2014. True to Leiderman form, my father and his attorney decided to flout the law and had not bothered to send me a copy of the testament, a requirement of California law for any heir-in-fact, regardless of whether they're named in the will. In exchange for my signature, I'd receive $25,000.

My attorney, who, like most people I met as a young adult around the greater Palo Alto community, was held in thrall by the fairy dust of my parents' Stanford affiliation and perceived status. Until that point, he had had a hard time believing what I told him about my family and my ostracism at their hands. His attitude was very much in keeping with what I've encountered when having to discuss any aspect of my father's activities with males of my generation.

In a disparaging phrase or two, they summarily dismiss the idea anything happened, slyly twisting the nuance of the discussion so my own legitimacy is called into question. Since it didn't happen to them, in other words, and it happened to a woman—me—the traumatic event is of no consequence and probably made up. The sentence is usually a variant of "I'm sure something happened, but I suspect there is more to the story."

With my father's deranged gesture, something finally fell into place. My father showed him exactly who he was. The attorney was stunned, in no small part because of the structure of California law. He could not believe the idiocy of the invasion, given the circumstances. California trust law was as unbreachable as the high-security wings at La Santé Prison in Paris. He knew, and he knew that I knew because he'd informed me himself, that there was no way I had any legal grounds to go after my parents' estate.

I didn't sign the paper.

Later, after I learned more about my father's death and the circumstances around it, I understood what had been so troubling to me during the month of March. My father, during his last weeks, was likely cursing my life. I had somehow survived his machinations and escaped. I had a talent he envied. How dare I? The rage and hatred emanated from California all the way to France, the way an airborne scent of rancid fat wafting from a greasy spoon miles away suddenly alights on the senses. Without being conscious of it, my preternatural antennae detected him.

Old and infirm, although still living at home with a part-time "personal assistant," when he really began to falter, my father was taken to the teaching hospital, where he had been a professor for thirty years. Within days of being admitted to Stanford Hospital, my father was transferred to the Palo Alto Veterans Administration Medical Center.

My sister indignantly described his transfer to the VA as a maneuver on Stanford's part to rid themselves of a "medically uninteresting" patient at the end of life.

I view this scenario rather differently.

Before she died, Andrea and I spoke several times a week. I flew out to visit with her and meet with her and her husband, Hayes. I wish we'd had more time. Andrea called me one day shaken, because of an encounter she'd had with her hepatologist. Andrea's primary cancer had metastasized to her liver. The tumor was the size of a baseball. Her hepatologist, a physician at Kaiser Permanente, had called her in to consult with her. He was furious. My father had phoned his practice, demanded to speak with him, and ordered him to locate a liver because he believed Andrea's life—which he'd done nothing but deride and devalue for forty years—could be saved by a liver transplant. I asked her if this was a possibility, and if it was, I'd gladly give her half of mine. She said it wasn't. Long before my father inserted himself, she and her doctor had discussed it between them: The mortality statistics for transplants for cancer patients were really bad.

"How bad is that?" I asked.

"One hundred percent mortality within a few months," she told me, trying not to cry.

"That's pretty bad," I replied.

But that wasn't what she was upset about. Her doctor, in high dudgeon, had castigated *her*, erroneously assuming she'd asked my father to intervene on my sister's behalf. He threatened to drop her and said he would not tolerate such a thing again. Having found myself on the wrong side of specialist doctors a few times when I had breast cancer—more than one medical oncologist who decried my refusal of chemotherapy comes to mind—I found the way he treated Andrea deplorable. That said, I'm sure he felt he was being disrespected. Andrea's self-important, Stanford-doctor father pulling rank on a local specialist doctor guy would not have sat well with any self-respecting professional.

"Did you tell him it wasn't your idea and that you knew nothing about it?" I asked.

"I did," she said.

"Did he apologize?"

"No."

"Can you find a new doctor?"

"No," she said, then cried in earnest. "It's too late. He'd already told me we were at the end of the road. No one else would take me."

I could barely contain my own rage.

To this day, I cannot come to rights with the torment my father caused her over the entire course of her abbreviated life, especially at its end.

The day my father was admitted to Stanford Hospital, he was the same man he'd always been: a weapons-grade malignant narcissist whose ascendant traits motored ahead full tilt, magnified tenfold by the knowledge he was losing control.

The COVID-19 pandemic had overwhelmed Stanford Hospital the same way it had the rest of the hospitals in the world. My father was not suffering from an acute and life-threatening case of COVID-19. He was, rather, a ninety-seven-year-old malignant narcissist in the grip of end-of-life collapse. His grandiose delusions about himself were unraveling. Medical staff were likely faced with a boiling lava pit of hostility, self-pity, and threats of dire consequences should they fail to comply with his orders. And this was during a worldwide pandemic unequal in scale to any other Western medicine had ever encountered.

As a private hospital, Stanford chooses whom they treat. The management elected to triage him out to a hospital that was both obliged to and probably better equipped to deal with him. They may have had more ancillary staff to deal with his outbursts. My sister D, who has never failed to make excuses for my parents' pernicious conduct—especially for my father, with whom she identified—saw my father as the real victim. The many burdens the COVID-19 pandemic placed on hospitals worldwide as a perfectly valid reason for his transfer did not exist for her. The COVID-19 detail did not count, except as her own excuse for not being at his bedside when he died. Stanford Hospital should have parted the waters for him.

"A distinguished faculty member just put out at the end of his life," she sniffled over the phone to me in Paris when she called to regale me with the details. I remained silent. She was and is my father's daughter, coxswained by her own narcissism.

At the VA, a caregiver saw him daily. He hallucinated wildly. There were dancing girls in his room. He was sure people were trying to harm him. At one point, something provoked him and he became, according to someone who had been present, "violent."

Rather than have an aide simply restrain him—I'd hardly think this would have been too difficult, given his age—and call his personal physician, who might have traced the source of the outburst to liver failure, the VA staff called security. For a while, security guards stood outside his door while the docs ignored him, perhaps as a kind of covert punishment for his behavior.

The end, as my sister described it, was more than a bit gruesome. The medical resident could not figure out that my father's liver had failed. Instead, he concluded that, since my father hadn't eaten or drunk anything for days, he must have been dehydrated. In fact, he was—so much so that his veins had collapsed and it was not possible to start an IV. So, the resident decided to intubate him. When he inserted the tube, he made the amateur's mistake and ran it down my father's trachea rather than down his esophagus. Or maybe it wasn't so much of a mistake. My father drowned in a few ounces of water.

My siblings' absence was noteworthy. My brother, a doctor himself in New Mexico, finally managed to get on an airplane, arriving on the scene shortly after my father's death.

Despite my feelings about him, it does not give me any satisfaction to know he was probably sad and scared at the end of his life. No children and no friends at his bedside to comfort him. What is the use of spending decades grooming your loyal offspring to be sycophants if they abandon you at the time of your death? My father died exactly as he lived: venal, vindictive, and alone.

Later, I sent Charlie an email consisting of a single sentence. "Your mother is prescient."

Charlie replied, "I assume your father just passed away? If so, my condolences. Please let me know if you have any more sightings of my mother."

I can't define the occurrences of the spring of 2021 in logical terms or even in metaphysical terms. To those who would say "they were a coincidence" or "they prove nothing about the existence of a metaphysical or transpersonal reality," I offer this comparison: I can't see the wind, and yet I know it exists. It demonstrates its presence in the way living creatures and inanimate bodies in the physical world experience and react to it: the fluttering of the leaves on trees, the pressure of a gale, and the sideways-sleeting rain. I can hear it whistle through Western canyons. Instrumentation can clock its velocity by measuring the rate of motion of the objects it displaces. It is known indirectly through its effect on the physical world.

The same could be said of gravity. I can't see gravity, yet I know it is there because all creatures of the earth do not float up into the stratosphere.

Recently, an intuitive I've been working with described my knowing ability as "claircognizance"—the innate ability to know things about people and who they are and to know things about the future.

It took me years to understand most others don't have this ability. I respond viscerally to people and am more likely to respond to interpersonal dynamics as they are rather than I am to respond to a preferred, often counterfeit, narrative.

To anyone who wants a more complete explanation for unseen or emergent phenomena, I offer this quotation from the play *Hamlet* (act 1, scene 5), where the protagonist addresses his friend

Horatio: "There are more things in heaven and earth, Horatio, / Than are dreamt of in your philosophy."

In the spoken English of 1602, *philosophy* meant what *science* means today—that magical incantatory word that men invoke when they are desperate to demonstrate their unique ability to sort and quantify what can be known of the world and its myriad processes through a narrow sliver of perceptual approaches known as "the scientific method."

CHAPTER 8

THE DARK SIDE
OF PSYCHEDELICS

It was always tempting for me to imagine that therapists of the psychedelic movement were going to be cut from better cloth than were those of my parents' generation. And yet they are not so fine after all. The cult of personality, the victim-blaming, and gaslighting in the field seem to be unkillable.

In the year following my first MDMA session, I began to comprehend what happened there in terms of the dimensions of what occurs in the psychedelic space when practitioners whose own drug use and persistent adulation by their clients and disciples lead them to believe they are larger than life. MDMA is an empathogen—a drug that produces feelings of emotional communion, oneness, and openness. Interpersonal boundaries can blur. In situations like these, the dangers MDMA poses intensify a participant's vulnerability exponentially. Normal rules of conduct appear not to apply. In retrospect, I now see that is what happened both during and in the days following my MDMA session at the Fischer/Meckel household.

Konrad's statement of his feelings of attraction to me ("I really like you"), along with Friederike's statement early in the session ("You're beautiful") as the drug effects came on unmoored me. I was supposed to trust them. Could I? I recall my thought at the time was, *I really do not need this.*

Even before the session, I had begun to feel as though the entire event had been engineered. Why ever did Friederike invite me? She was busy with her therapy clients, which left Konrad to take me under his own wing. Their intentions seemed less like selfless gestures toward a woman on her own in a Parisian COVID-19 hellscape than as a balm to relieve themselves of their own ennui. Confinement was boring. My visit was a welcome diversion.

As the week went on, the lingering effects of the drug session colored the time I spent at their household. On several mornings, I engaged with Friederike in integration sessions during which we sat at a table and she encouraged me to examine my feelings about our role-play in which her daughter played the part of my mother. But the MDMA session and its aftermath seemed to serve as a kind of blind over the dynamics occurring in her own household.

Konrad surprised me one evening when I was emerging from the sauna in the basement. I was naked and about to shower. Suddenly, there he was. Seeing him approach, I told him I'd just gotten out of the sauna. I pulled a towel off a hook and wrapped it around myself. He halted, stared at me unflinchingly for maybe thirty seconds, then turned and went back upstairs. This encounter engendered some longer-term fallout.

The couple's own backstory is one of manifold boundary violations.

After her first marriage ended, following an affair from which she emerged devastated, Friederike began Holotropic Breathwork training, among many other therapeutic modalities, to help her on her quest to confront her own issues and eventually use her knowledge to help others. Konrad came to her as a client. He, too, was divorced. She taught him how to practice Holotropic Breathwork and introduced him to MDMA.

The two fell in love. Friederike's daughter (who was in our MDMA session) later left her own husband to marry a former client of Friederike's, who was also in the session. His former wife, who was also a one-time psychotherapy client of Friederike's, was the client who had outed them to the police over a decade before, blaming Friederike for the breakup of her marriage. Konrad and Friederike both spent time in prison for illegal possession of a small quantity of LSD and paid hefty fines. Konrad gave up his license to practice law as a result.

Their casual air toward holding an MDMA session in their home, given their history of problems with the law, astonished me. (And why in the world would they include a woman they'd never met before?) Although nothing physical or aggressive occurred, the boundary violations took a toll. They brought up feelings from my childhood, of having been used as a pawn in my parents' alcohol-infused *folie a deux*. I had often been separated from my siblings. I felt, once again, that I was back at home in the worst possible way. I found myself revisiting the wished-for idea of home as a place of safety from the outside world.

I did not write about these occurrences, initially. I, too, succumbed to that all-too-intrusive rationalization process many have described when finally reporting bad experiences with psychedelics: I didn't want to believe it was true; I did not want to harm the "psychedelic movement."

Now I have other thoughts. I don't want evangelistic zealotry and all-too-common ego inflation, which skews the judgment of many practitioners within the psychedelic movement, to bring further harm to vulnerable patients—and particularly to women.

Once the Paris lockdown was over, I moved to Alsace to get my bearings and to have the contents of my house delivered to me, finally, from storage, so I could sort through them prior to my now-two-year-delayed move back to the United States.

Living within a few hours of Konrad and Friederike, I suggested a visit. Over the course of the year, I asked them a few times if they would meet. I suggested to Konrad that we meet for coffee, as a way of clearing the air. Each time, I was rebuffed. They no longer spoke to me. I would have expected psychedelic therapists—or any therapists—as experienced as they would be more self-aware about their own issues, and their own boundaries, and be able to face them.

Not so. I was especially troubled by Konrad. Once I'd made my own boundaries clear, we spent what were for me pleasant hours together walking and talking in the forest above the town with Konrad and Friederike's dog Yago, who, unsurprisingly, had boundary issues of his own: stealing food from the table and counters; grabbing tissues from my hand; tearing up furniture when his owners were away from home. Trained for years by a professional dog trainer, Yago's expensive schooling would fall to pieces each time he was returned home after a tune-up.

With Konrad, I was able for the first time to speak candidly and openly about my marriage, which had ended in 2005. He was thoughtful and reflective. Knowing I used to ride horses, he'd taken me to the barn where he rode. He invited me to take a few lessons, if I liked, on his own horse or on another horse in the barn. He invited me to a hotel he owned in the mountains for a night—an experience whose boundaries I made a point of defining and clarifying explicitly with him in advance of the excursion as non-intimate and social only. He seemed fine with my candor—at least on the surface—protesting that he was able to have women friends and had many, his riding instructor among them.

In the end, the scenario with Konrad and Friederike evolved very differently from that of my first psychedelic experience. I feel as though I was used as a toy. My vulnerability and isolation, my very reasons for trusting them when I was literally at my worst, were my weakness.

I now feel as though I made an error in judgment because of my own needs. Even so, I can't discount the benefit I got from the role-play during the session. I am no longer trying to save my four-year-old self. She's saved. We're one person.

As a result of that session, I now question whether MDMA is the right drug for female trauma survivors, especially when guided by practitioners who have boundary issues themselves. There's the rub: How is one to know in advance? The inflated self-image many practitioners project, refined over many years, coupled with a sense of their own infallibility, often becomes mixed up with their own unacknowledged needs. They're not likely to be doing much self-examination. Boundaries become even more porous under the influence of the drug because of the flood of oxytocin it causes and the feel-good messages it can elicit when participants take it together during the session.

MDMA for veterans is a different story because of the nature of their experiences and the nature of the population itself. In general, male veterans as subjects are coming to grips with guilt and shame over *what they did to others* during war in service to an outside authority.

Many—not all—did not relinquish their own agency, even if they chose to submit to the demands of the service hierarchy. Their autonomy and their own power never actually failed them, unless, for instance, they became prisoners of war. I was told by a man who was sexually molested in his early teens by the director of his summer camp that his experiences left him feeling he'd lost his autonomy. It's taken him his entire life to overcome his PTSD. His experience as a male who was sexually abused by a man when he was a child gave him the sad ability to know on a visceral level what women undergo when they are being victimized by men.

Women dealing with sexual, physical, and emotional trauma must come to grips with their internalized shame and fear because of *what was done to them when they were powerless*. Many traumatized women relied for their survival on their abusers, whether they were parents, guardians, or spouses.

MDMA compounds our vulnerability. Under the influence of MDMA, women relinquish personal agency, as we were forced to do when we were abused. Under the drug, we are entirely powerless. Guides or therapists who are willfully unaware of their own boundaries certainly have no regard for ours.

In the years since my experience at the Fischer/Meckel household, I've taken part in other MDMA sessions and subsequent sessions with ayahuasca and psilocybin under the guidance of an entirely different kind of practitioner, a woman who is highly regarded for her competence, both in Switzerland and in the United States, where she often travels to run psilocybin sessions for people suffering from terminal illness. Her expertise is such that the university hospital in Zurich retains her to train doctors to conduct psychedelic sessions as they prepare themselves for the entry of psychedelic therapy into the world of clinical medicine. Working with her has redressed some of the harms done by my first MDMA experience.

I now believe the classic psychedelics are much more suitable for women dealing with trauma when used with the right guides in the right setting. MDMA should be avoided altogether, unless the guide is a close friend and has intimate knowledge and understanding of the scope and depth of the emotions women with PTSD can experience during sessions.

Now, though, a humanistic priority is unlikely to prevail around psychedelics. Any notion of collective good has been supplanted by the unbridled and insatiable greed of profiteers in the psychedelic space.

The True Cost of Psychedelics

During the past few years, the evangelical fervor around the introduction of psychedelics as a potential treatment for depression as well as for other emotional and neuropsychological disorders (OCD, smoking, PTSD) has catapulted enthusiasm for these drugs miles ahead of any considerations of their downsides. There are many. This trend has been driven largely—in the United States, at least—by the burgeoning involvement of pharmaceutical investors determined to make a killing by turning psychedelics into the next go-to pills for all manner of ailments. In their mania, these players are willfully ignoring the dangers psychedelic and entactogenic drugs present in clinical settings.

The questionable use of psychedelics in Western medicine has a long and checkered history, starting with mescaline, then LSD.

In the mid-1950s, Dr. Jean Delay, president of the Faculty of Medicine at Centre Hospitalier Sainte-Anne, conducted an experiment in which he and a colleague gave intravenous infusions of LSD-25 to seventy-five mentally ill patients, seventy-two (96 percent) of whom were women.[1]

The purpose of the experiment, ostensibly, was to study whether LSD-25 could be useful in therapy as an aid in eliciting memories of highly charged emotional experiences from childhood. In particular, Delay's professed motivation for the experiment was to see if LSD-25 could enhance the process of "transference," in which a patient unconsciously projects feelings originally felt in childhood onto the analyst. Among Freudian psychoanalysts, transference was commonly believed to be a key to a successful analysis.

Delay described the women as "cases belonging to an economically modest environment and of a cultural level that is often the most undeveloped."[2] The women, in other words, were neither educated nor sophisticated. Delay did not provide any editorial commentary about the men. None of the subjects were given any information about the medication, although it became clear during the experiment that at least some of them—despite their lack of sophistication—had figured out there was a hidden agenda. The patients had a diversity of diagnoses, among them chronic delusions, schizophrenia, delirious episodes, postpartum depression, anxiety, nervous depression, obsession, psychopathy, dementia, and melancholia.

Delay designed the experiment so that there were times when the subjects were in an office with an observer and times when they were alone. The point of the experiment, Delay wrote, was not "reporting a complete study of the reactions under LSD-25, such as one could obtain in volunteers, but of exposing what can be acquired in practice . . . with minimal intervention of the observer."[3] In other words, the patients were not "volunteers." They were unwitting recruits in a drug experiment.

The observers, doctors, and assistants under Delay's charge were discouraged from interacting with the subjects. They were there to watch and take notes. The patients experienced the onlookers' detachment in various ways.

"What a spectacle I'm giving you," said one woman. "I must look stupid, disheveled. I feel diminished, ridiculed, I don't know how much to take."[4]

Another said, "You stay there without moving without any human gesture. Instead of comforting me, you do nothing. You are there, dry, severe, like my father."

Several of the women felt they were being mocked.

One implored the doctor not to make fun of her. "I'm begging you, it's not funny. I can see very well they laughed at me. It must be funny to be questioned."

Seven of the women figured out they were the subjects of an experiment. Said one, "They come to observe us."

Another said, "Studying my case that isn't understood very well, we are the guinea pigs, we're in service to others afterward."

Someone else said, "I would not want to sleep. I would be scared that you would do something to me."

Seven women felt they were being tortured. "Everything around me is hostile, I have nothing familiar. Do not torture me anymore," said one.

About a subject who was obviously having a distressing time with the hallucinations and stood up for herself, Delay wrote, "She protests during the experience, despite having been warned in advance."

Warned of what, exactly? Delay does not specify. Perhaps she and the others in her group had been told the injection may cause unpleasant side effects. But it is clear the woman felt she'd been tricked.

She demanded to know, "Why have you done this to me? You don't have any right."

Delay noted, somewhat mockingly, "She criticized us because 'she was not asked for her permission.'"

Zoë Dubus, a doctoral candidate in contemporary history at Aix-Marseille Université and a researcher associated with the Institut des Humanités en Médecine and the Centre Hospitalier Universitaire Vaudois, Lausanne, Switzerland, tried to find out who the women were so that she could make contact with them. She hoped at least a few would be alive and willing to talk. She was unable to contact them. The hospital would provide no details about them.

"We don't know anything about them, the pathology, whether they were married, or whether they had children, whether there are surviving relatives. They were an accumulation of numbers," said Dubus when I spoke with her.

Although the records must exist somewhere in the bowels of the hospital, archiving systems are either nonexistent or else well-hidden to prevent anyone from finding anything out.

"One woman was seventeen when she was admitted," said Dubus. "She could still be alive or her relatives or children could still be alive."

Dubus tried to communicate with an archivist at Sainte-Anne, who told her simply, if they don't have the name of the patient, they can't even start to locate the file.

"They were not motivated to try to locate the files and the names. I don't know whether they don't have money for someone to go through and catalog them or whether they don't want those files to be made public."

Dubus attributes the attitudes of the doctors to the general attitude of the medical profession at the time, which in some ways still endures in France.

"The idea of 'care' is really new in France. In the profession here, empathy is lacking. It's a vertical approach. The expert doctor speaks and declaims. The patient does what he is told."

The Anglo-Saxon tradition is very different.

"In England, habeas corpus law applies. Patients can be heard in justice if they are treated unfairly," said Dubus. "They have individual rights that can't be subsumed under the will of the doctor. In the United States and United Kingdom, doctors listened because they could be sued in law if they did not listen to needs of patients. In France, doctors are really like gods. They don't have to listen to patients," explained Dubus.

That said, things did change somewhat in 1997, in theory at least. A case came before the Cour de Cassation (France's highest court) in which a doctor performing a colonoscopy perforated the patient's colon, leading to a peritoneal infection and emergency hospitalization. The patient sued on grounds of not being adequately informed of the risks of the operation. He had argued in a lower court that he could not prove he had not been informed because he had not been informed enough even to know there were risks he should ask about. The case eventually advanced to the high court and the patient prevailed.[5] The court's decision overturned long-standing precedent in French medicine where it was simply assumed patients had no rights, and doctors' status made them above reproof.

Moral responsibility of the doctor in the context of inpatient care at Sainte-Anne aside, Delay's stated scientific goals for the LSD study—how LSD could serve the Freudian holy grail of "transference" (results published in the journal *Éncephale* in 1958)—belie a cloaked agenda.[6] Evidence shows that in the mid-1950s, Delay was under contract to the French Ministry of Defense in a project designed to ascertain the usefulness of LSD as a tool for enhanced interrogation of prisoners of war, as well as a pharmaceutical aid for mind erasure.

A document dated February 20, 1956, refers to a "visit to the Hôpital Sainte-Anne" by a representative of the Sécretariat Permanent of the Comité d'Action Scientifique de Défense Nationale (the permanent secretary to the Committee of Scientific Action of the Ministry of Defense) where studies relating to the "psychic conditioning of prisoners of war" were discussed with Delay.[7] These, according to the file, could be addressed in two ways: through animal studies, which "demand the establishment and maintenance of large and expensive animal facilities," and through "trials on humans, whose infrastructure (premises, materials) is much less expensive and could possibly be carried out at Sainte-Anne." The studies, continues the report, could be relatively simple, particularly since a number of such studies had already been carried out on Sainte-Anne inmates on the effects of "amphetamine shock, glutamic acid, narcotics, and the effects of mescaline and LSD-25 (parallel to those at the School of the Americas)."[8]

A subsequent file dated June 8, 1956, titled "Sections: Human Problems [and] Biology" and "relating to psychochemistry" makes explicit the interests of the United States.

Several doctors, including Delay, were consulted on the topic of "products to facilitate deconditioning and reconditioning in the context of psychological warfare." Their report was handed over to a Commander Gordien, who, according to orders, "should pass it on to the Scientific Attaché of the Department of Defense in the USA."

Although Delay was never explicitly associated with MKUL-TRA, the Cold War CIA program whose mission was to develop enhanced interrogation techniques as well as techniques for reprogramming the human mind, someone he came to know in the context of studying the effects of psilocybin indeed was.

In 1956, Dr. Roger Heim, director of the French Museum of Natural History and director of the laboratory for the study of mycology and tropical phytopathology at the École Pratique des Hautes Études in Paris, accompanied businessman and amateur mycologist Gordon Wasson to Oaxaca, Mexico, to collect psilocybin mushrooms. The expedition, Wasson's third, was clandestinely funded by the CIA under MKULTRA Subproject 58.[9] The funds were offered to Wasson by an undercover CIA officer to underwrite his research following his so-called discovery of psilocybin mushrooms on an expedition the year before in the town of Huautla de Jiménez.

On returning from Oaxaca, Heim extracted psilocybin from mushroom samples he had cultivated at the museum. Then he consulted with Delay. The two concluded that psilocybin was a good candidate for experimentation on the inmates at Sainte-Anne. Wasson's wife, pediatrician and expert ethnomycologist Dr. Valentina Pavlovna, observing the positive mood effects of the mushrooms, advanced the idea that psilocybin could be beneficial as a therapeutic tool. Lab-grown mushroom samples were sent to Swiss pharma Sandoz, which refined the drug to its active component, psilocin. Sandoz provided sufficient medical-grade psilocin for subsequent experiments on inpatients at Centre Hospitalier Sainte-Anne.[10]

The first experiment was less a therapeutic undertaking than a psychomimetic exercise: Observe the responses of mentally ill and healthy subjects while they are under the influence of drugs to determine what, if anything, changes.

This study was carried out and supervised by a young psychiatrist, Dr. Anne-Marie Quétin, as part of her doctoral dissertation in 1959. Psilocybin was administered to twenty-nine healthy volunteers and seventy-two mentally ill patients. Among the healthy volunteers, twenty-four subjects were men, five were women, all of whom had "an average or higher sociocultural level," according to the doctoral dissertation describing the experiment.[11]

In the mentally ill group, eight were men and sixty-four were women. The medicine was presented to these subjects as "either a means of release or as a complementary experiment necessary for diagnosis." They were not told about the drug's mind-altering effects. Their knowledge about the experiment and the drug they were receiving was inadequate. However, they received slightly better treatment than the LSD-25 subjects. They were referred to by name rather than number in published records, and their personal stories mattered enough that the investigators actually knew who they were.

There was one bright spot in this medical undertaking: On April 20, 1959, a thirty-five-year-old inpatient named Henriette B received the first of two intramuscular injections of eight milligrams of psilocybin to treat her anorexia nervosa.

Henriette B was the first person to receive psilocybin to treat anorexia. Henriette B's response was initially successful. She started eating and gained weight. But her recovery was fleeting. She regressed once she returned home to her family and was subsequently readmitted. With each readmission she improved only to deteriorate again when she returned home.

Instances of patient abuse and torture using psychedelic drugs to further the Cold War agenda of mind control under the umbrella of the CIA's project MKULTRA are well documented.

Among these were experiments conducted by Dr. Donald Ewen Cameron in the 1950s and 1960s at the Allan Memorial Institute of McGill University in Montreal in an experiment he conducted with funding from the CIA. Cameron admitted patients with relatively minor mental health issues, such as anxiety or depression, into his hospital's inpatient wing. Patients were placed in medically induced comas, given LSD, and compelled to undergo electroconvulsive therapy. Cameron said his experiments would cure his patients' illnesses by erasing certain memories and reprogramming their brains. But many of the patients were unable to return to normal life after their treatments. It turns out that the "deconditioning" part of mind control is a lot easier than the "reconditioning," just as tearing down a building is a lot easier than building one.

The MKULTRA program was shuttered in 1973. This did not halt medical and therapeutic malfeasance in psychoactive drug experiments.

When Zealots Helm the Ship of Scientific Inquiry

The end of the Cold War marked the official cessation of involuntary psychopharmacological experimentation with psychedelics on human subjects. For about thirty years, during the psychedelic-drug prohibition era, there was no above-board science done with psychedelics at all. When clinical trials resumed, first with MDMA in 1994, the profile of the participants was entirely different. Informed subjects were eager to be admitted into the studies. One would think the study design and the fact that the subjects weren't being used as unwitting laboratory rats would have made the modern clinical trials unassailably safe. Alas, it was not to be so.

Recently, clinical trials sponsored by MAPS have gone seriously off the rails. The sexual abuse of a woman patient during her MDMA session revealed a sea of iniquity. Revelations about how MAPS had conducted clinical trials soon made the news. Rick Doblin, the organization's head and chief executive, has been advocating for the legalization of MDMA as a therapeutic drug since the 1980s. As of this writing, Doblin is sixty-eight. His unalloyed devotion to his MDMA crusade at the expense of any and all other considerations has called his ethics and the integrity of his fanatical pursuit of legalization into question.

Several women came forward to tell their stories about what they experienced during their MDMA sessions in a podcast produced by *New York* magazine.[12]

Each of the women subjects had undergone a similar series of three MDMA sessions with two professional therapist guides over a span of three months.

According to more than one of the women, the first sessions were "amazing" and allowed them to process traumatic memories.

"Everything was revealed," said one subject. "I went chronologically backward and unloaded all the traumatic experiences."

"It was like peeling back a curtain. . . . It was going to be okay. I felt like I was going to make it," said another.

Things began to unwind after the second session.

One subject said she felt "wide open and unresolved after [my] second experience." She began to understand the danger of the territory they were leading her into. She emerged from that second session terrified and feeling hopelessly dependent on her therapists.

By the time the last session rolled around, she dreaded the study's imminent termination.

"I contemplated gluing myself to a chair until they agreed to continue seeing me," said yet another.

Several experienced similar feelings. One said she felt as though she was "begging [the study therapists] to find a way not to kick me to the curb."

One compared the experience to having open-heart surgery, where the surgeons walked away from the table mid-surgery, leaving the patient's chest cavity gaping open, her heart exposed. "No one is going to survive that," she said.

All of these subjects suffered from PTSD; they were childhood sexual abuse survivors, childhood physical abuse survivors, or rape victims. All of them bought the hype propagated by MAPS.

If they trusted and believed in the therapeutic process, all would be well.

In any area of life, this belief system is called "magical thinking." Sometimes characterized as a form of delusion, magical thinking is a perceptual system in which thoughts, beliefs, and certain actions are believed to influence or control real-world events, sometimes despite huge evidence to the contrary.

Besides the psychological and emotional damage left by incompetent therapeutic support during and after sessions, MAPS was discovered to have suppressed data that did not suit their agenda. In Phase 2 trials, placebo outcomes were often superior to drug outcomes. These results were not reported.[13] MAPS reportedly consistently jettisoned study data that did not serve the company's interests, such as data from before- and after-session questionnaires, where women who were not predisposed to psychotic symptoms reported having psychotic episodes after their MDMA experiences. Temporary psychosis was one of the many reported side effects of recreational MDMA.

The volume of overlooked or dismissed data has called into question the validity of the MAPS Phase 2 trial dataset.

As Lily Kay Ross, one of the coproducers of the *Power Trip* podcast, pointed out in the podcast: "You can only catch the things you measure."[14]

It is clear, from the information that has become public, that MAPS made studied decisions about which outcomes they were including and which they were discarding. What were they looking at, and when did they deliberately avert their gaze?

One of the MAPS Phase 2 clinical trial subjects, Meaghan Buisson, was sexually abused during her MDMA sessions in 2015. She took part in a MAPS study conducted in British Columbia, Canada, by Richard Yensen and Donna Dryer. Yensen himself was not a licensed therapist and should not have been conducting sessions in the first place. Buisson obtained a video recording of her session from a MAPS employee.

After the videos of Buisson's sessions were made public by *New York* magazine, Health Canada ordered a review of all further MAPS clinical trials in that country.[15]

Further patient-safety issues led to the suspension of one of the two Canadian clinical trials for MDMA-assisted psychotherapy underway in 2022.

Doblin is neither scientist nor doctor. His background is in political science. He has devoted his entire career to his personal obsession: the legalization of MDMA as a medical drug. He has never done anything else. The dawn of his advocacy began with experiences he himself had with drugs and those he witnessed among friends when he was in his twenties.

During the course of the revelations about Buisson's experience, Doblin could not have demonstrated less concern about the consequences for the injured woman. His contempt for the study subjects who blew the whistle was barely veiled. Like the Freudians and experimenters before him, he immediately turned the assault back onto the victim, claiming, in an interview, "Her inner healer should have been able to guide her on how to respond."

The fact that the tape shows a pinioned Buisson on a bed, thrashing frantically and shouting, "Get off!" from beneath the burly Yensen, who weighed easily one hundred pounds more than she, seemed to escape Doblin's notice. Dryer, the second therapist—and Yensen's wife—stood beside the bed, clownishly pressing Buisson down.

Doblin's response echoed that of Yensen, who, when defending himself in a civil lawsuit brought by Buisson in 2018 in a British Columbia court, turned the blame for the assault back onto Buisson herself, labeling her "a skilled manipulator."

In psychiatry speak, "skilled manipulator" is a code phrase, a portmanteau word hauling along with it diagnoses of "borderline personality disorder" and "hysteria" as not-so-subtle suggestions the victim is, because she is a woman, "crazy" and therefore herself at fault for what the therapist did to her.

A number of men in the psychedelic movement dismissed Doblin's idiotic response to the Buisson tapes, growing defensive when asked to account for the new psychedelic doublespeak embodied in the phrase "protected by the inner healer."

The psychedelic movement as it has taken shape in the past half decade is dominated by privileged Caucasian males. As a group, they have no interest in addressing misogyny. Instead, they rocket happily forward while the culture distills and refines the abuses and, at the same time, denies them, adding a new age twist of sadism, veiled by insider's privilege. The message is the same, however: *We're the psychedelic he-men, and you're a woman. We own this space. Whatever happens to you here, you entered of your own free will. You're responsible for your own abuse.*

As of this writing, no one from MAPS has defined the term "inner healer."

The many MAPS subjects who reported on their abuse felt his response compounded their victimization. Several women study participants were asked if they could identify the mysterious "inner healer" who purportedly leaps onto the scene during MDMA sessions to protect them from sexual assault by the therapist. None could, and none had any idea what this phrase was supposed to mean. None of the therapists, when queried, could offer a definition.

Perhaps not coincidentally, when Doblin began lobbying the FDA for approval of MDMA as a therapeutic drug, he targeted veterans as the first and most promising cohort for his new treatment modality.

According to Doblin, "It was a large, easily identified group that was generally found to be sympathetic to a broad range of people."

Yet there's a bit more to it than Doblin's simplistic statement about this select group: Almost none of them are women.

A cohort that is 99 percent male, trained in combat, and easily able to defend itself against attackers presents a distinctly different profile than do women PTSD sufferers. In the study setting, where subjects are under the influence of an oxytocin-producing, psychological-boundary-disrupting drug, a woman dealing with sexual or childhood trauma is more physically and emotionally vulnerable and faces an entirely different set of risks than those faced by a male ex-Marine.

Women are far more likely to be taken advantage of in therapeutic situations. This fact is well documented. But for men with narcissistic traits and ego issues like Doblin, women represent an Achilles' heel that can fell the army of true psychedelic fanatics. The fact that they might have something to say about untoward sexual behavior of men with whom Doblin identifies throws in a variable that someone such as he would not want to confront. To him, it's the women in such a situation who are the real danger: They're the Bouncing Betties.

The so-called Bouncing Betty was an antipersonnel land mine used widely during the Vietnam War. Buried at a depth of a few inches with a three-pronged trigger hidden by vegetation, the mine detonated when one of the prongs was disturbed. The mechanism would launch itself upward to waist level, where it would deliver a barrage of ball bearings and shrapnel, killing and maiming victims up to 460 feet away. The Bouncing Betty was known for its psychological effects on troops because it was more likely to inflict debilitating wounds than kill its victims outright.

There are serious problems with fanatics like Doblin determining the course of scientific endeavors and running clinical trials. Scientific research, at its core, was designed to avoid situations like those created by MAPS. Medical ethicist Emma Tumilty, a lecturer at Deakin University in Melbourne, described the situation as akin to the church peddling holy water.

"If the Catholic Church was going to set up a bunch of trials to tell you how holy water was efficacious for doing something, we would all take those with a pinch of salt," said Tumilty in an interview with Lily Kay Ross and Dave Nickles for an article in

New York magazine.[16] Whether they were motivated by money, or belief, doesn't really matter. "I'd like somebody else to do that study," said Tumilty.[17]

Doblin lacks many crucial qualities needed to carry out credible scientific drug research. Among the most central is impartiality. There should be no inherent bias and no agenda about whether the drug under study will work. Investigators must be as open to the idea of total failure as they are to unambiguous success. Scientific objectivity and detachment from outcomes have been woefully absent from the fields of psychiatry, pharmaceutical drug development, and, more recently, psychedelic drug research. Doblin's forty-year record of unalloyed fanaticism, coupled with his lack of an ethical gyroscope, disqualifies him from engagement in any kind of medical drug research at all.

Doblin, however, is undeterred. Asked during an interview by Ross and Nickles what it would take to derail a drug trial with MDMA, Doblin replied that only a substantial number of suicides would cause him to call the safety of the MDMA studies into question.[18]

CHAPTER 9

THE CULTURE IS THE MEDICINE /
THE CULTURE IS THE POISON

$$\diamondsuit$$

*Culture is the primary vehicle for delivering healing.
The overarching principle articulated by several [Native
American] healers interviewed was "culture is medicine." Connecting with one's culture has both protective
and therapeutic value, promoting both resilience to and
recovery from traumatic events.*[1]
　　　　—DEBORAH BASSETT, Ursula Tsosie,
　　　　　　and Sweetwater Nannauck

It did not take me long after I moved to the United Kingdom in
2009 to realize that the depression that followed my diagnosis
of breast cancer had little to do with the cancer. It had to do with
leaving the community and country where I felt safe and was
known, of which I was a part, in order to pursue medical treatment
that I no longer had access to in the United States. I had to leave

because of the sadistic economic agendas of the neoliberal political class, which had become synonymous with "America" over the preceding forty years, a movement that has annihilated the notion that any life has meaning if the capital class can't profit from it. Neoliberal ideologues have taken over the political, commercial, and social reality in the United States and the United Kingdom. There are no signs they're slowing down.

I recall the day in 2009 I told some of my classmates at Columbia Journalism School, where I was on a one-year fellowship in science journalism, about my diagnosis. I didn't know word had already gotten around. A young South Asian classmate, Aman Sethi, a brilliant writer and raconteur, suggested we go for a walk. We traversed the Columbia campus and headed out the Amsterdam Avenue gate toward Morningside Drive. He'd determined the best balm was a recounting of the Sanskrit verse scripture the *Bhagavad Gita*, which consists of a battlefield dialogue between a prince, Arjuna, and his charioteer, an incarnation of the Hindu god of protection and compassion, Krishna, about the morality of fighting a war in which one knew one would slaughter lots of people, including many relatives. Aman began by explaining how radical the idea was when it was composed, that there was more than one "right path" to spirituality and enlightenment. Aman asked if I knew anything about the *Gita*. I didn't. He told me that it was only one book of the Sanskrit epic the *Mahabharata*, which contained hundreds of narrative threads, each layered into the next like the sedimentary rock formations found in the western United States and on Mars. As we walked toward Morningside Heights, he laid out the plot of the *Gita* and its place in the *Mahabharata*. Each substory, he pointed out, contained seeds of the next story, and it didn't really matter in the course of the telling whether the first story or the second came to a resolution or not. Each story unfolded fractally, like Mandelbrot sets opening up all the possible events in the universe before our eyes.

When we returned from the walk an hour or so later, I was in much better spirits. I realized even then that something I had here sustained me, and to leave for the sake of medical treatment would cause any sense I had of belonging to this community in New York to vanish. I'd soon lose touch with the friends and acquaintances I'd made in the six years since I'd left California.

I'd be starting over again, only this time, in another country. It would be even worse.

Once I arrived in England, I refused all the oncological interventions pressed upon me by National Health Service doctors. They were determined to persuade me I needed chemotherapy, which I'd already turned down in the United States—both because I couldn't afford it and because I had read the scientific papers and understood the numbers. The doctors insisted surgery and radiotherapy alone were inadequate. They disdained my informed understanding of the phrase "7 percent chance of recurrence." With each successive annual examination, NHS breast docs gnashed their teeth and insisted I at least keep the appointment they were required to make with the next medical oncologist, who inevitably would call into question my decision not to undergo chemotherapy. They seemed horrified that I understood the odds of my cancer returning or metastasizing to another location within five years of my diagnosis were less than the odds of my being hit by a drunk driver while crossing the road in London.

My climb out of the bog of the American health system was probably not worth it. If I had to do it over, I'd throw myself on the mercies of the New York State welfare system.

Data have shown in study after study that the most important factor in healing from any emotional, neuropsychiatric, or actual corporeal illness is the presence of a cohesive and functioning community surrounding the person who has either lost their health or lost their way. Community is the reason so many twelve-step fellowships are successful.

This fact of human nature—the need for community and interdependence—also demonstrates why the placebo effect in medicine is so powerful, especially when it comes to psychedelic medicine. The support provided by the interactions with the guides and the medical staff heals trauma more effectively than the drug. Any drug. Naturally, the existence of the placebo effect is a tremendous inconvenience to those who peddle pharmaceuticals, like MAPS, for instance.

In clinical trials with MDMA, study subjects who received the placebo also received all the guidance and support they would have received had they been given the active dose. MAPS found the subjects' vastly improved emotional states to be an unsavory truth, for its purposes, and dismissed placebo data, declaring sniffily, in published literature, "Current trials are not designed to evaluate this question."[2]

When I returned to England following my second Hopkins session, I was more than depressed. I felt I had nothing to look forward to. My emotional state was evident to the Hopkins researchers when they called to follow up. Roland Griffiths, the principal investigator, and Mary Cosimano, the study coordinator, suggested I return to Baltimore, where at least they'd be able to provide some support. I pointed out that I still could not get medical care in the United States, and I still did not believe Obamacare would last longer than one administration. Although they professed great concern about my well-being, I felt that their interest in the state of my feelings had less to do with compassion than it did with the study dataset. If I were to attempt suicide, Roland would have had to declare me an "adverse event." Roland's research sponsor, the Heffter Foundation, which had paid for my trips to Baltimore from London, would have to accept that my participation was a wash. My experience could not be included in the data presented as evidence in the case for the efficacy of psilocybin to treat depression. Roland could not have counted me among the success stories and used my experience to bolster further applications for research funding. That's how the academic machine works. The study would be considered successful only if it could be used to leverage the next one. If I had, in fact, attempted to end my life, the data collected about me and my experience would have been pulled from their publishable results and entrenched into some other category.[3]

My fate was unimportant. The real concern was damage control on behalf of the mission of proving, according to the increasingly ludicrous dicta of the twenty-first-century scientific establishment, that Roland's and the other researchers' beliefs about psilocybin were unpuncturable and irrefutable and nothing that happened could change them.

I refused to seek psychotherapy, even though I'd agreed to start swallowing SSRIs at some point, long before I started in the study. In the United Kingdom, SSRIs are often prescribed to breast cancer patients along with the medical treatment. Yet I knew from the get-go the problem was not *inside me* and no amount of jabbering to a therapist was going to fix it. SSRIs sure didn't. The problem was that I had no one, and all I wanted to do was go home. Antidepressants weren't going to cure me of "not belonging," nor was anything else. No amount of personal erasure could turn me into someone who fitted into an old, closed culture of which I was not part.

After considerable prodding from Roland and Mary, I did eventually find some therapeutic support through a breast cancer charity in Fulham in West London that offered, among other things, a few free sessions of Reiki therapy, courses in mindfulness meditation, and meetings with a financial advisor. Her advice was probably the most useful of the lot. She guided me through the benefits offered by the council and various charities now that my income was severely reduced. Hopkins also provided monthly conversations with my session guide, Fred Reinholdt. After about six months, I started to get my feet under me.

In 2013, my former husband in California finally settled accounts with me, leaving me with enough money to purchase a tiny bit of dirt I could call mine. So, in 2014, with the European Union squarely in the crosshairs of the St. Petersburg–manipulated

British neoliberals and Brexit looming on the horizon, I decided to move to France, where, I had learned, property was much cheaper. And there was more room. My decision to move to France represented my attempt to treat my life like a business. That method of making decisions by itself was probably a mistake.

In 2015, I bought a cave house outside of the town of Tours in the Loire Valley. The house, which I loved, was tucked into the side of a limestone cliff beneath a little wood and vineyard. It made me feel better. A huge wisteria plant climbed up the front face. I planted climbing roses. A little flock of bats whooshed in and out of one of the caverns every evening. Eurasian wrens, *Troglodytes troglodytes*, cave birds, made their nests in limestone crevices. There were hedgehogs, seasonal hoopoes, lizards, a species of broad, flat toad, cuckoos, and Eurasian blackbirds. I was still very much an alien, despite having added UK citizenship and legal permanent French residency to my collection of identity papers, because I'd failed to carry out the first and most obvious maneuver expected of any single woman who wishes to conform: Find a male of the right age and wrap herself around him like a strand of ivy.

The physical fact of my house provided much solace. I spent my time reading, walking my dogs, and writing the occasional article. I created a garden. I watched birds. I observed the night sky. I ran a summer guesthouse in one of the finished cavities in the complex of caves where I lived, called a *gîte*. People came and went: Australians, Chinese, Americans, and Germans on bicycles were among the most memorable.

In 2017, after learning of our mother's death, I'd begun a cautious contact with my sister, D. We moved gingerly toward figuring out whether we could have a relationship, given what had happened in our childhood.

In 2018, D and her husband came to visit. We met for lunch in Azay-le-Rideau. I identified safe topics in advance: birds, food, dogs, the weather, and French history, about which I know nothing. My brother-in-law, a big fan of the intrigues of the château-dwelling French aristocracy, was a veritable font of information.

One night a few months after their visit, I sat in the domed cavern of my living room bundled in blankets on the sofa with a fire blazing in the woodstove. I found myself gazing into a psychic space I call the Void. The dogs lay on the sofa beside me. A motherless baby Eurasian blackbird I'd rescued a week before was sleeping in a box in my bedroom. The light from the fire and the candles on the mantel flickered against the uneven scoring on the softly curving limestone walls, creating a vision of an animate universe; within the walls, birds, lizards, and mice were moving in and out of limestone shadows. Then the domed ceiling was replaced by the dome of night sky in the Sierra Nevada foothills where I'd lived when I was married.

I found myself contemplating the yawning gap between the time I'd left my family of origin behind and the present. What was the nature of those relationships, whose slender filaments still seemed to tether me to the world?

I found myself in my father's suburban Boston office, more than fifty years before, in the middle of the night, the night I'd raised my voice against my abusers and told them I hated them. The regular, dotted, grid pattern of the asbestos ceiling tile so popular in those years replaced the textured mattock-scoring of my cave walls. What had made me able, on that of all nights, to resist them and their violence, to scream out and to defend myself? What power imbued my words so that my own voice actually stopped my parents' fists mid-blow?

I look back and see a presence, something not quite embodied.

For a while, as a child, I told myself a story of an angel. I could comfort myself with the odd wish that there was an angel out there, somewhere, looking out for me. I held it out as a kind of goal to look ahead to. If there were an angel, then there might be a future. All I had to do was figure out how to survive.

The journey that night continued. I made my way again under the winter night sky; the constellations and the Milky Way were visible overhead. Then there was total darkness. I had the sense of making a choice, as though I was being asked if I wanted to continue or if I wanted to stop and turn back. I kept on, not knowing where I would end up, how I would end up, or whether I would be alive at the end of the night. The darkness was as inviting as velvet. Rather than finding a place to be feared, I found in the Void a place of dark, encircling welcome. Then, like an arm outstretched across my path, something stopped me, and I was back in my own domed living room with guttering candles, the once-roaring fire now embers. A dog was snoring. Light was creeping in the window. The baby bird was shrieking from the bedroom. Now wide-awake, she had to be fed.

Comforting as my cave house was, hiding out with dogs and a baby bird wasn't really a life.

On the outside, life in France was hell. From the day I'd moved into my cave, I'd been harassed and threatened by a deranged neighbor who felt I should not be allowed to use my deeded right-of-way past his mother's house up to my property. He threatened me with hedge clippers, slashed my tires, and left his shit outside my gate. Police came; reports were filed. But in France, there are no anti-harassment laws. Under French—Napoleonic—law, in order for such an assault to be brought before a judge, I would have to be found dead, or maimed, or be able to show proof that the neighbor himself had done the damage to my bodily person. Then there could be an inquest.

A woman on her own in France has few rights. A woman of foreign birth on her own can be ground into the dirt and no one will notice.

I grew increasingly scared and stressed each time I drove up the lane to my house. The mayor of the village, a peroxided member of the local aristocracy, the daughter of a local *caviste*, a kind of person locatable in what is known as *la France profonde*—deep, rural France, where foreigners ought never to stray unless they're wealthy wine collectors—provided no support, implying that I, as an interloper, shouldn't expect the cadastral laws to apply to me. It didn't matter that the right-of-way had been settled in a lawsuit thirty years before and that it was mandated by the court. I was just a foreigner.

"Vous êtes en France maintenant, Madame Rex!" she shouted out the window of her black Mercedes one day, chastising me as she sped by for disposing of my trash in a town skip, which I was doing only because I was afraid to wheel my bin down my own lane, fearful of imminent assault by the neighbor.

After five years and the mounting conviction that modernized and well-maintained cave houses like mine were going to be forced into compulsory purchase by her and the local government, if not immediately then within the next few years, I put my beloved house up for sale in early 2019.

In January 2020, the preliminary sales contract was signed, and I happily went to New York, where I planned to find a place to live, once the house sale was finalized, in June.

Then the COVID-19 pandemic hit. In mid-March, I had to rush to get back to France before the border closed.

The Culture is the Poison

The COVID-19 pandemic threw into sharp relief just how toxic Western society has become, from the early falsehoods spread by both government and media about the seriousness of the new virus to the gaming of the availability of protective gear to forcing people to return to jobs where they were all but guaranteed to contract the illness. In the United States alone, the total number of deaths from the mishandling of the COVID-19 pandemic over the course of three years from January 2020 until April 26, 2023, was 1.13 million.[4] Compare this figure with the Second World War. During the entirety of the US engagement, from December 1941 until the 1945 bombing of Nagasaki, 405,399 US military personnel lost their lives.

The trajectory of the COVID-19 pandemic enabled some of the more rapacious players in the psychedelic world to unmask their true colors. What unfolded was an almost surreal display of preening and strutting narcissism by men who are now the self-proclaimed leaders of the movement.

In the last decade, an entirely new kind of human has taken over the psychedelic scene. They could not be more different from those I encountered when I took part in a clinical trial over a decade ago at Johns Hopkins and from the movement's primogenitors: María Sabina Magdalena García (the Mazatec *curandera* who unwittingly provided psilocybin mushrooms to businessman and CIA operative R. Gordon Wasson in 1955), Timothy Leary, Alexander and Ann Shulgin, and Dr. Walter Pahnke, to name a few.

The work of bespectacled—and biased—academics like Roland Griffiths has been engulfed and overtaken by a group of neoliberal profiteers who could not have demonstrated less commitment to social welfare, the common good, and civil society if they'd rolled in on tanks and thrown those asking for help with their life issues into pits.

The "entrepreneurs" like Christian Angermayer, a German investor, founder of the investment firm ATAI Life Sciences, are emblematic of the predatory male creature who has emerged in the last few years, fueled with cash and obsessed with the goal of dominating the psychedelic world.

Angermayer's psychedelic origin tale goes like this:

He "discovered" magic mushrooms while on a cruise with friends on a yacht in the Caribbean. In another version, he went to the Netherlands to a retreat and tripped in nature. There's a version about Malta. Or was it Papua New Guinea? With each new version of his story, he's reassured his audience he ingested the drug in waters or time zones that made his activity entirely legal, preparing his audience for his own version of the new reality: He and he alone would dictate the future of psychedelics. And it would be pharmaceutical. His insights were typical of the grandiose crew taking over the psychedelic space. Rather than envision how he could help humanity at a calamitous time, Angermayer's epiphany consisted of a singular vision of himself making a killing medicalizing psilocybin and marketing it at a premium as a medical treatment for depression. He himself, he protested, never suffered from depression. He's a clear-eyed capitalist, merely pursuing a hot business opportunity in a world that values this skill above human life itself.

Since his fateful first trip, Angermayer has become the world's largest psychedelic pharma investor. The company he's staked his future on is Compass Pathways, now a publicly traded pharmaceutical company based in Britain. Compass is in the business of cornering the market on medical psilocybin through various insalubrious yet creative methods and deals, such as patenting psilocybin, a naturally occurring substance which has been in use for several thousand years. They are also attempting to patent elements of the therapeutic process itself: the layout of the therapeutic chamber, and when and how the guide touches the patient during the sessions.

Angermayer displayed his loose relationship with both facts and truth as well as his utter contempt for the humanity of anyone who is not part of his privileged neoliberal ilk in the many tweets he issued during the early months of the COVID-19 pandemic. Among the most telling was a tweet of March 18, 2020, quoted on the website Psymposia, in which he protested against a complete lockdown to forestall further life-threatening disease transmission. "To go on with complete shut down for more than 2 wks is absurd and violating any civil rights we fought for. . . ."[5] As one of the new poster boys for psychedelic capitalism, he appeared confused about what civil rights were and who was entitled to them. To him, workers were nothing more than disposable, vulgar peasants who must toil away to enrich him in the midst of the ravages of the worst pandemic since the arrival of HIV/AIDS.

To suggest they have either civil or human rights *themselves* would no doubt come as a surprise to him.

"The idea that we must prioritize 'economic health' over public health ignores the reality that, under late stage capitalism, 'economic health' is actually code for elite prosperity, which does not translate into greater individual or societal health," wrote editors of the website Psymposia in a post from April 2020.[6]

What was it psychedelics were supposed to do for people? Oh yes, demonstrate the true meaning of life, open our hearts with compassion for others, and reveal the unity of all living beings. Wasn't that it?

Here's the rub. One of the most glaring dangers of psychedelics is their tendency to amplify existing personality traits, including grandiosity (or Machiavellianism) and narcissism. Where traditional societies once selected leaders from among those with the most life-affirming and alliance-building personality traits such as agreeableness and conscientiousness, over the last forty years or so, the rise of neoliberalism has created the perfect climate for the growth of dark-factor traits such as greed, sadism, narcissism, psychopathy, and grandiosity. Corporate culture and the neoliberal economic and political policies that have swept both the United States and the United Kingdom since the late 1970s value these traits above all others, adding fuel to an already-out-of-control cultural and sociological conflagration. We see the results of it everywhere, from rising poverty and homelessness to illiteracy to violent crime to environmental degradation to the climate catastrophe. Add psychedelics to the dark-factor-trait explosion, and these once hallowed and sacred substances become vehicles of endangerment—not for the persons who have ingested them but for everyone else.

An extreme example of this effect was Charles Manson, a hallucinogenic drug user and criminal cult leader whose followers carried out several high-profile murders in Los Angeles in the late 1960s. The most notable was the murder of Sharon Tate, the wife of movie director Roman Polanski.

Angermayer learned the same lesson as all those others whose grandiosity and egotism were amplified by the psychedelic experience—a frighteningly common occurrence among privileged males. And there's no moderating force stopping him, no ritual process, no ethical backbone, no religious heritage, no built-in shame, no complex and interdependent community that creates social norms and expectations about the common good. He's the embodiment of late-stage capitalism, of the coming fascist machine and its total disregard for life, human or otherwise. Imagine someone such as he understanding with humility and compassion that community well-being is more important than whether he makes a million bucks today. Or any day. Perhaps psychedelics should be made available only to cultural groups that use them ceremonially and therapeutically, or to religious groups that use them as sacraments. They're simply too dangerous in the hands of the neoliberal capitalist class. Imagine a neoliberal operating without an ego. I cannot bring such a thing to mind. Providing psychedelics to men such as these is like handing a shiv to the person who has promised to murder you.

The Psychology of Neoliberalism

Neoliberalism and narcissism have been on an interlaced upsurge in Western culture since the end of the Second World War and especially since the 1970s. Perhaps it's no coincidence that this trend correlates with the suspension of military conscription in the Western, educated, industrial, rich, and (supposedly) democratic world, which broadly speaking includes the United States, western Europe, and Britain. It also correlates with the end of a postwar era when the common good was fairly widely accepted to be more important than the accumulation of infinite wealth by a small set of culturally and socially privileged individuals who have benefited in ways never before seen in the Western world from extreme neoliberal economic policies.

The only institution in Western society that fosters cohort identity among adolescents is the military. There hasn't been a military draft since the Vietnam War. The last day of the US draft was June 30, 1973. The book *The Culture of Narcissism* by Christopher Lasch was published in 1978.

Although believing in the necessity of going out and killing a perceived enemy does not make a better human out of anyone, one of the most important features of military service is the highly ritualized process of basic training that generates group cohesion among (primarily) young men. It's an initiation rite.

Using forced austerity and pushing the limits of physical and psychic endurance, basic training, my former husband, a Vietnam War veteran, once said (I paraphrase) "teaches any snot-nosed asshole of a kid with an attitude what is important so that he'll never forget it as long as he lives."

Every soldier learned—some for the first time in their lives—he was responsible for his buddies' survival. Your platoon mate dies, it's on you.

Does the absence of a culturally mandated initiation explain the explosion of narcissism among Western males over the last fifty years?

This sideways slide away from any consideration of the common good is typical of neoliberal psychology, according to a paper published in the *Journal of Social Issues*.[7] The authors list the characteristics of neoliberal psychology, which I paraphrase here:

1. A radical abstraction of the self from place and time—that is history—as well as from social and material context, including choices about creation and dissolution of both individual and community ties.

2. The invention of the entrepreneurial self—that is, the cultivation of an externalized [ego-driven] self—to create and extend a marketable brand.

3. A commitment to growth, which includes freedom from

obligations, expectations, and norms, and an emphasis on self-expansion and personal fulfillment.

4. Control of affect—that is, suppression of feelings and control of emotions—substituting high-arousal positive affect (excitement, optimism, enthusiasm) as an index of health and morality key to success.

That these same tendencies form much of the psychological makeup of psychedelic drug users comes as no surprise.

In the United Kingdom, researchers interviewed twenty magic mushroom users to ascertain their feelings about psychedelic drugs within their cultural context.[8] They compared the subjects' drug use to the way psychedelics were used in the 1960s. The study found there were two overarching themes. The first placed the participants' discussions squarely within neoliberal rhetoric. They characterized themselves as rational, risk-managing persons engaged in a form of "calculated hedonism that was legitimated as an act of personal freedom and consumer choice." The second both celebrated and problematized a collective, connected "hippie" or "post-psychedelic" form of spirituality.

None of the subjects viewed their choice to use psychedelics as anything but an expression of free will. They were unable to imagine a world in which they considered the good of the collective as a primary, superseding virtue that influenced how and in what way they made personal decisions about taking drugs or doing anything else.

THE CULTURE IS THE MEDICINE

In the early 1990s, medical anthropologist and associate clinical professor of psychiatry and human behavior at the University of California, Irvine, Dr. Marlene Dobkin de Rios collaborated with Dr. Charles Grob on a project to explore hallucinogenic drug use in three communities where psychedelic substances are an integral part of near-universal rituals marking a young person's passage from childhood to adulthood: Australian aborigines of the Central Desert Region; the Chumash of Central California; and the Shangana Tsonga of Mozambique. They compared the use of hallucinogenic substances as part of the ritual process with the pattern of drug abuse among American adolescents at the time.[9]

Drug-abuse patterns among young people in the United States and Europe, they noted, corresponded with a pattern of dysfunctional family life, accompanied by dysphoria and self-medication. Here, the use of plant medicines, including tobacco, as well as alcohol and other mind-altering drugs, has long been dissociated from any meaningful cultural context.

Drug use in Western society over the last forty years tracks with an increasing sense of alienation in the middle class since the end of the Second World War, paralleling the breakdown of extended families, community, and a general sense of continuity, cohesion, and belonging once provided by a thriving cultural tradition.

Hallucinogenic plant consumption by young people in indigenous tribal societies often occurred as part of a ritual initiation process. A young person just starting puberty enters into a liminal or marginal state; then endures a days- or weeks-long series of physical and mental challenges; then emerges as a changed person, now prepared to participate in adult society, with all of the responsibilities and privileges that entails.

The Chumash Indians of the Santa Barbara, California, region used a preparation of ground *Datura meteloides*, known locally as jimsonweed or *toloache*, in their initiation ceremonies. A skilled practitioner, the *tolachero*, prepared and administered the drink to the young initiates.

Datura meteloides, if consumed as is in flowering form, can cause fatal seizures. Whoever prepares it must have a thorough understanding of the plant and how to prepare it.

The young men were given the *toloache* when they were considered strong enough to withstand its powerful psychedelic effects, a few years after puberty but before they were sexually experienced. Five elders, "givers" of the substance, gathered in a boy's house and administered the potion. Boys were told to pay attention to the dreams they experienced while intoxicated. When the initiate awoke, he was sung to and instructed to see beyond surface appearances and to "receive an animal spirit helper like a Hawk or Coyote to offer him lifelong protection and guidance.[10] After the intoxication ended, the Datura givers asked what he had seen in his visions, which they interpreted. "The elders 'moralized,' and in the youth's heightened, hyper suggestible state, they were able to inculcate culturally important moral systems and values."[11]

The most important feature of the initiation rite among all three non-Western cultural traditions that Grob and Dobkin de Rios studied was the creation of an intense, several-day ritual process within a cultural milieu where young people learned to sublimate their individual needs and drives to those of the greater community. They write:

> These states were created to heighten learning and create a bonding among members of the cohort group . . . so that individual psychic needs would be subsumed to the needs of the social group. This was done to ensure survival. Cohort identity might be fostered by the austerities and painful consciousness changes that accompanied genital mutilation, sleeplessness and beatings—a sort of aboriginal boot camp—where one would share and identify with one's cohorts upon whom survival success might often depend.[12]

The reverence for transcendence and unity created by transitional ceremonies, and with it the lessons imparted to initiates during altered states of consciousness—such as codes of ethics, the veneration of the common good, and a sense of cultural continuity—has been lost in Western society. Psychedelic use outside of activity promoting spiritual growth has denatured the significance of these substances and the lessons they impart. Instead, it has become one of the many available anodynes used to fill an existential emptiness, devoid of values found in communities where the human soul once thrived.

The União do Vegetal Church: Ayahuasca as Sacrament in a Modern Community

Over the last fifty years or so, a few institutions have quietly incorporated the psychedelic ritual tradition into a cultural and spiritual practice. The Centro Espírita Beneficente União do Vegetal (the Beneficent Center of the Union of the Plants, or UDV), is one of them. Founded in Brazil in the early 1960s by José Gabriel da Costa (Mestre Gabriel, as he came to be known), a rubber prospector working in the Amazon rainforest, Mestre Gabriel became acquainted with ayahuasca when he participated in ceremonies with the rubber-gathering indigenous and mestizo populations working along the Brazilian border between Bolivia and Peru.[13]

Da Costa returned to the settlement of Rio Branco, having had a spiritual awakening in which he envisioned transmitting a message of peace to the world. He gathered a group of followers and created a structure and mythology for his new religion, a syncretic church whose elements of evangelical Protestantism, baroque-folk Catholicism, and afro-Brazilian religiosity as well as of indigenous cultural and mystical tradition reflected the diverse heritage and complex colonial history of the area.

As part of the religious sacrament, UDV members participate in church rituals using ayahuasca a minimum of twice monthly but often as frequently as several times a week.[14] The UDV requires its membership to abstain from all other psychoactive substances, including alcohol, tobacco, marijuana, cocaine, and amphetamines.

By the mid-1990s, the UDV had grown to about seven thousand members in Brazil. The adherents were highly diverse, hailing from both rural and urban areas, and included people from across the ethnic, socioeconomic, professional, and educational spectrum.[15]

As of this writing, the UDV has a presence in ten countries: Australia, Canada, Italy, the Netherlands, Peru, Portugal, Spain, Switzerland, the United Kingdom, and the United States.

Ayahuasca, or hoasca as it's known in Brazil and within the UDV, is a tea preparation brewed from two psychoactive plants, principally the bark of the vine *Banisteriopsis caapi* and the leaves of *Psychotria viridis*, a shrub that is a member of the Rubiaceae or coffee family. *Psychotria* contains approximately 0.3 percent dimethyltryptamine (DMT) as well as other alkaloids, such as beta-carbolines and *N*-methyltryptamine. The DMT in *Psychotria*, when ingested orally, is broken down by the digestive enzyme monoamine oxidase, which inactivates its hallucinogenic effects. Monoamine oxidase is counteracted by the *Banisteriopsis caapi*, a flowering vine that contains the psychoactive alkaloids harmine, harmaline, and tetrahydroharmine. Harmine and harmaline are monoamine oxidase inhibitors. When *Banisteriopsis* and *Psychotria* are drunk together, the harmine and harmaline prevent the digestive system from breaking down the DMT in *Psychotria*, allowing the characteristic intense DMT hallucinations to proliferate. Tetrahydroharmine is also a psychoactive substance, akin to psilocybin in that it binds to the same neuroreceptor as serotonin, inhibiting its reuptake. It is also known to stimulate neurogenesis, which accounts for the reports of improved memory among UDV members.

Hoasca use throughout the Amazon and Orinoco basins has been part of cultural ritual practice for at least a thousand years. Hoasca was used ceremonially to induce altered states wherein indigenous practitioners communicated with the spirits of their ancestors, envisioned detailed enactments of mysterious occurrences, and made contact with supernatural entities, often embodied in visions of jungle forest animals like serpents or jaguars.[16] Hoasca was also considered medicine, used by practitioners both to diagnose and treat illness.

Folk healers in the mestizo populations of the Amazon basin administered hoasca to selected groups of patients, adhering to the shamanic models practiced by aboriginal peoples to bring about divine or ecstatic states and as means to access realms of the supernatural.[17]

In Brazil, the UDV church operated with little interference until 1985, when the constituent plants were added to the list of banned drugs. The church filed suit against the government of Brazil, challenging the law. After an investigation, the Brazil federal drug council concluded that hoasca-using church members were healthier and more productive in their communities than the average citizen.[18]

In 1993, following the lifting of the ban, the UDV invited a multinational group of researchers to Brazil to study the psychological and biochemical effects of their tea. Having an objective, scientific study in hand could protect them, they reasoned, if the political winds were to shift once again.

The study was conducted in Manaus, where the oldest UDV congregation outside of Rio Branco was located. The researchers recruited fifteen members of the UDV from a large group of volunteers, all who had been ritually drinking the hoasca tea for more than ten years. A control group of fifteen was also recruited. The experimental subjects ranged in age from twenty-six to forty-eight years. Two had been born into the UDV. The others had been members for ten to eighteen years.

Many of the subjects reported having been engaged in a variety of dysfunctional behaviors prior to joining the UDV.[19] Eleven had been addicted to alcohol prior to joining; two had been jailed for violence. Four were abusers of other drugs, including cocaine and amphetamines. Eight were addicted to nicotine. Several described themselves prior to joining the UDV church as impulsive, disrespectful, angry, aggressive, oppositional, rebellious, irresponsible, alienated, and unsuccessful.

Each subject described transformations in their lives as resulting from their experiences with the ritual use of hoasca within the context of the church. Many of them felt they underwent a life-changing perceptual transformation during their very first ceremony.

A common theme in describing their altered states was visions of total destruction—of being in car wrecks, on unstoppable carousel rides where getting off was impossible, of being attacked and dismembered by ugly wild animals—unless they changed their lives. Many reported encountering a vision of Mestre Gabriel, who would deliver them from the terror.

Subjects reported that, since joining the UDV, their lives had objectively changed. Besides quitting whatever substances they may have used, they "emphatically stated that their daily conduct and orientation to the world around them had undergone radical restructuring."[20]

Said one subject, "I used not to care about anybody, but now I know about responsibility. Every day I work on being a good father, a good husband, a good friend, a good worker. I try to do what I can to help others . . ."

Others stressed the importance of practicing good deeds, watching one's words, and having respect for nature among the many lessons they'd learned. Many reported improvement in memory and concentration and continual positive-mood states, a sense of fulfillment in day-to-day interactions, and a sense of meaning in their lives.

Among the most striking results, though, was the universal understanding of context in the efficacy of the sacramental use of hallucinogenic substances:

> They saw the hoasca as a catalyst in their psychological and moral evolution, but were quick to point out, however, that it was not the hoasca alone that was responsible, but

rather taking the hoasca within the context of the UDV ritual structure. Several of the subjects were in fact quite critical of other Brazilian groups which utilize hoasca in less controlled and less focused settings. Subjects described the UDV as a "vessel" that enables them to safely navigate the often turbulent states of consciousness induced by hoasca ingestion. The UDV is their "mother . . . family . . . house of friends," providing "guidance and orientation" and allowing them to walk the "straight path" . . . The subjects also emphasized the importance of "*uniao*," or union, of the plants and of the people.[21]

Many subjects criticized other Brazilian groups for using hoasca in uncontrolled or casual settings. Of all the observations made by the UDV members who were interviewed, one in particular stood out: their comprehension of the dangers of hoasca without the structure of the UDV.

Without it, hoasca experiences could be unpredictable and *lead to an inflated sense of self.* This observation has been shown to be universally true. Within the Western neoliberal tradition, the inflated self is now out of control.

Magical Thinking About Psychedelics is Not the Solution to Ourselves

The psychedelic movement has revealed an essential truth about healing: The collective, supportive, spiritual, and ritual aspects of the psychedelic experience in community settings are what relieve suffering and strengthen ties. I would love to imagine that those who make policy about the delivery structures in medicine and mental health treatment would opt for a course of action where the former model becomes a backbone of medical practice and community mental health. The trend, however, is headed unremittingly in the opposite direction. These decisions, along with every other public policy decision, are now effectively made by resource-extracting, profit-obsessed companies whose executives do not care about the human condition any more than they care about the well-being of any living creature or, for that matter, the well-being of the planet. Every structure in place enables and abets this system, from pharmaceuticals to insurance to education to transportation to natural resource management. Western culture ruled by the unbridled narcissism of *Homo sapiens* businessmen and a mechanistic, profit-driven relationship with the natural world threatens physical health, mental health, and life on earth.

It doesn't have to be this way. Just ask those who know a whole lot about plants.

In the 1980s, anthropologist Dr. Jeremy Narby, working in the Peruvian Amazon, learned about the ways of a tribal group called the Ashaninka. He described them as people "who know a lot about plants and animals. . . . They have a name in their language for just about every species living in the forest," said Narby. Their reverence for and intimacy with the natural world was conveyed through the way they spoke about plants and animals: as beings with characteristics, values, and purposes. "They even called some species Ashaninka, which was their word for themselves, meaning our people or our relatives."[22]

Narby described in an interview a conversation he had with a young Ashaninka ayahuascero trainee. Narby asked him how he had come to know about plants. The young man explained to him that the only way to learn about plants was to drink the hallucinogenic brew made from the vine. It was the plants themselves who could teach him about plants. No one else could do it.

Saving us from ourselves will require a paradigm shift, a way of looking at the world in which things that grow and things that animate, relate, inspire, and teach are more important than things that turn a profit. We will start having to listen to the plants and to each other. The all-important concepts of "maximum productivity" and "maximum return on investment" will go the way of the punch card reader and the buggy whip.

I do not know whether humanity will survive long enough to learn how to learn from plants or to become as intelligent as the plants are. If we do, we may have a chance of saving ourselves. As of this writing, I'd call it a long shot.

EPILOGUE

SEEING WHAT IS THERE

In 2022, I returned to the United States after living abroad for thirteen years. Since I landed at Dulles Airport a little over two years ago—two suitcases, two dogs in two crates, two passports, one UK, one US, a *carte de séjour permanente* (France), a *carte vitale* (also France), and no place to live—I have been trying to make sense of what has happened in this country since my departure.

I chose to enter the country via Dulles Airport outside of Washington, DC, because I knew if I flew into JFK, the chance of my being reunited with my dogs within a few hours was remote. Dulles was reputed to be straightforward when it came to accompanying animals. And so it was. My dogs were delivered in their crates to the baggage claim area and were waiting for me when I arrived.

But in the baggage claim area, something was terribly wrong. Most of the people milling around looked as though they were suffering from jaundice. The color of their skin was off—grayish, yellowish where it should have been pink. The number of young people whose faces were mottled with acne was astonishing. There were no individual luggage trollies. By the time I managed to make my way out to the curb with the dogs, where a driver was scheduled to meet me with an SUV, I could not stop crying.

The complexions were but one emblem of what American corporations have done to the populace. The overwhelming prevalence of obesity is another. There is little in the way of real food from farms available at most stores here because the agricultural and food-processing corporations want it that way. People have become addicted to factory food, with its added chemicals, high-fructose corn syrup, salts, fats, and augmented flavors. The architecture of such an economy is nihilistic by design.

My first encounter with the American medical system in fourteen years spoke volumes. Before I even entered an exam room at a general practice office in Kingston, New York, I found myself in an altercation with the business staff—a small army in charge of billing who demanded an up-front payment of $150, in case my insurance (now Medicare) proved inadequate.

In the exam room, I was unable to comprehend why it took three layers of personnel to do simple tasks all doctors in France do themselves.

In France, there are no nurses in doctors' offices—not even those of high-toned specialists—and office staff consists of one person to do the scheduling, if that. Sometimes a part-time staffer takes care of billing details that fall outside of the usual *Securité Sociale* (*la Sécu*) protocol. Most GPs do it all themselves. They answer their own phones.

Nurses are professionals in their own right. When not employed by a hospital, they have their own practices and provide a distinct set of services, such as blood draws, home health visits, health checks, and vaccinations.

Here, an aide changed the paper on the exam table and another aide took my temperature and blood pressure. A third person, the nurse, entered and began asking me a spate of questions. Following a few questions about my menstrual history and number of pregnancies—I demurred on that one—she asked, "How many live births?" I thought I'd heard her wrong. She repeated the question. A chill ran down my spine.

"I've never been asked that question before, not by an internist, not by a gynecologist, not by anybody," I said.

"It's part of your medical history," she said curtly. "You have to answer."

"I have no obligation to answer that question. It's no one's business, not yours, and not the medical staff." Her gaze narrowed.

The United States is the first country in the developed world to go on a rampage against women's rights. The foremost among these is the right to legal and safe abortion. Was this some kind of *Handmaid's Tale*–inspired medical plot to track and persecute women who had undergone abortions in the past? Given what had been happening in some states where abortion had been banned and where vigilante groups were allowed to hunt down women traveling out of state to seek care, I wondered what they planned to do with the information.

I was then seen by a nurse practitioner from Ukraine. Despite her relatively genial manner, I could not wait to get out of there.

It was for this reason, among others, that I decided to return to France in September for a follow-up lung scan. A small medical snag had emerged a few months before I was scheduled to leave France the year prior. A lesion showed up on a thoracic scan and, because I'd had breast cancer, my GP sent me to a pulmonologist, who ordered a biopsy. The results showed a bit of scar tissue, nothing more, but a follow-up in a year had been highly recommended.

Over the time I spent in Paris during the lockdown, I'd become acquainted with some of the people involved in psychedelic research in France.

Among them, researcher Vincent Verroust, cofounder of the Société Psychédélique Française, the French Psychedelic Society, has been an invaluable resource and has become a good friend. Vincent is engaged in the arduous task of moving psychedelics from the list of banned substances in France to the treatment room, particularly for treating obsessive disorders such as alcoholism.

Besides its charter to shepherd the reintroduction of psychedelics into the clinic and reform public policies on narcotics, one of the society's activities is offering monthly online integration circles "to allow people who have had disturbing, indecipherable, or painful psychedelic experiences to find a space for expression, sharing feelings, and engaging in collective discussion in a spirit of self-support," according to their website.[1]

Vincent has been experimenting personally with psychedelic drugs for many years. He's probably the most sophisticated and knowledgeable psychonaut I know. Lately, he's focused on DMT and 5-MeO-DMT.[2] Among the many virtues of these substances, which include, according to research, stimulating neuroendocrine function, immunoregulation, and anti-inflammatory processes, they have been shown to promote both neuroplasticity and neurogenesis in mice.[3] In other words, they can have a sustained positive effect on brain function, which, if translated to humans, could be very promising for a variety of maladies, including dementia and Parkinson's disease. In addition, 5-MeO-DMT also has a profoundly positive effect on anxiety.

Having suffered throughout my life from anxiety, which became extreme during the lockdown, reaching a point of such severity I developed heart palpitations and had to undergo a cardiac workup, I was willing to give it a try. My original psilocybin session had helped, to be sure, but it was not definitive. Especially since the pandemic, I'd been more anxious than ever. The move back to the United States and the challenges I'd encountered precipitated even greater anxiety.

DMT and 5-MeO-DMT are both ingested as inhaled vapor. A tiny amount of crystalline powder is put into a vape pen, heated to a high temperature so it evaporates, and the vapor is then inhaled. The chemicals are absorbed by the alveoli, rapidly enter the bloodstream, and are taken up by neuroreceptors in the brain.

I decided to try DMT and 5-MeO-DMT for myself. As the planned evening approached, I began to feel a great deal of trepidation. The substances themselves, DMT and 5-MeO-DMT, are very different. I'd drunk DMT as ayahuasca tea on a few occasions with a guide from Zurich when I was living in Alsace during my last year in France. It promotes highly visual hallucinatory experiences that are, in many ways, similar to those of psilocybin. The hallucinations have their own logic and their own narrative. Although they can be intense, they are nothing like what happens when one inhales 5-MeO-DMT. Of all the common hallucinogens, 5-MeO-DMT is considered among the strongest, producing an experience of complete ego dissolution for most people, which is not always the case for many of the other serotonergic hallucinogens, such as psilocybin, LSD, or ayahuasca. The experience of total ego dissolution often results in better outcomes for those seeking relief from depression and anxiety.

A guide arrived in the evening with the accoutrements. They'd cued up music on a laptop. They asked me several times to check my blood pressure to make sure it was stable. Both DMT and 5-MeO-DMT could promote sudden fluctuations in heart rate and blood pressure. In France recently, a man with an undiagnosed heart condition suffered a heart attack and died during a pseudo-shamanic session where he was given large amounts of psilocybin mushrooms and 5-MeO-DMT within a short space of time. My blood pressure, like my heart rate, was predictably low. I do, however, suffer from asthma, and I wanted to take a puff of asthma medication before we started. My guide was not keen on this because the active ingredient, albuterol, tends to increase heart rate for a minute or two. I complied, despite the fact I saw no cause for worry.

Both DMT and 5-MeO-DMT in their crystalline form were provided.

Although DMT is a scheduled drug in France, 5-MeO-DMT is not.

It was decided I should try the 5-MeO-DMT first, and then the DMT. I was not so sure. I'd spoken at length with others about how 5-MeO-DMT takes effect and what it does.

Inhaling these substances is unlike ingesting normal doses of psilocybin or ayahuasca. The onset is instantaneous, like being shot out of a cannon or, as I came to experience it with 5-MeO-DMT, being shot out of an airlock into outer space. The experiences last from ten to thirty minutes, even though they can feel as though they last an eternity.

The DMT effect sounded a lot like ayahuasca. I thought I'd try the DMT first, then see how I felt. As I always do before going on a psychedelic journey, I spent a few minutes before I started contemplating my emotional state and formulating an intention, a sense of some insight I wanted to gain through the experience. My emotional state was anxious, heightened by my trepidation about the effects of the drug itself. My intentions had to do with community and connection, which I felt I had lost since I left the United States in 2009 and which I felt were now unattainable in the fractured country I'd stumbled into. I reentered my country of origin with what emerged to have been false hopes: that my remaining siblings would have become people other than who they actually turned out to be—not, in other words, authoritarian personalities reenacting the hell of our parents' creation—and that the country would resemble a place I recognized. I had questions, and there did not seem to be answers.

When I was ready, my guide handed me the vape pipe with the DMT and instructed me to inhale, hand them back the pen, hold the vapor in my lungs as long as possible, and lie down. I inhaled and started coughing.

DMT, in its powder form, is most often an extract distilled from hallucinogenic indole-alkaloid-containing plant material, such as *Mimosa tenuiflora* or *Psychotria viridis*. The organic matter makes it much harder to inhale for those with compromised lungs.

But I managed to inhale enough for long enough for it to have some effect. I immediately arrived in a space where I felt I was underwater. Indistinct figures moved about. Then, Lord Ganesh appeared.

The Hindu deity Ganesh has a human body and the head of an elephant. He is known as the guardian of thresholds and the lord of new beginnings. He embodies symbols of success, enlightenment, and divine energy. My favorite Ganesh feature is his rat. Ganesh is often depicted riding atop a rat as he traverses the universe. This noble steed, the indefatigable rat, can chew through anything, thus symbolizing Ganesh's ability to destroy obstacles. Ganesh is one of my heroes.

The experience was brief—less than ten minutes—and I was soon back in the room. My guide thought I should try another dose, which I did, but it proved too caustic for my lungs, and I could not hold my breath long enough. Then, after several ambivalent minutes, as well as taking two tablets of L-theanine, which the guide had brought with them to help reduce my anxiety, I agreed to try the 5-MeO-DMT. The 5-MeO-DMT would be less irritating to my lungs, the guide assured me, because it was lab-formulated and contained no organic matter whatsoever.

They handed me the vape pen.

The moment I took the first puff, brain-piercing music like that of glass chimes or an antiquated musical instrument I have since managed to identify as an armonica surrounded me. The strains were far from mellifluous, the notes simultaneously harmonic and jangling. Whence it came, I could not tell. It was accompanied by a blinding light, which enveloped the room. The rhythm of the music choreographed itself with the frequency of the light waves, creating an eerie sense-bath that increased in amplitude with each passing second. As the intensity increased, the physical world began to come apart. The last recognizable thing I saw was the disintegrating image of my guide in the now-disintegrating living room as they reached for the vape pen, ordering me to lie down. Supine, I tried to breathe into the experience. Then the ceiling and the walls fractured into a blinding, tessellated pattern, resembling tiles of a Persian mosque styled not in azure and turquoise hues but white on nacreous white, radiant light emanating from between them, while the music—at times so agitating and penetrating it was like listening to fingernails being dragged across a chalkboard—engulfed me.[4] Above me was a mosaic dome of light. The music induced a sense of motion, like rocking or swaying. I lay back, feeling slightly seasick, rendered helpless by the bombardment, and yielded to the sensation that sound and light were united in some kind of numinous mission.

Then suddenly, the light was gone, and I was in a void, a volume of curved space, suspended . . . by what, from what, I had no clue. I was afraid. There was a bit of motion, like a ripple on water, and I thought, *Oh there might be life here.* But I was uneasy. Then, a small face appeared in the upper-right corner of my visual field. It was that of my friend, neuroscientist Mona Sobhani, who had tried 5-MeO-DMT as part of her exploration of psychedelics following an existential crisis wherein she discovered she no longer could conform to the dogma of scientific positivism demanded by her profession.[5]

She said, "You have to let go."

I've never been sure what this phrase means, but somehow, some element of my pneuma unclenched its grip on my notion of reality. And suddenly I was not there.

To be both being and not being is almost impossible to describe.

The experience was radically ineffable. There was a place, but it was not a physical place, and it was also not an emotional place. There was no color—or the color was darkness. I was, simply put, the universe. The universe and I were indistinguishable from one another. I did not see anything, I did not feel anything, and I did not know anything. I had no field of vision. There was nothing to observe. I had no sense of the passage of time or of a context. I was. The universe was. Nothing else mattered. Then I noticed motion, this time a sense of orbital movement, like electrons revolving around a nucleus or planets orbiting a star. The magnitude of the motion, whether molecular or interstellar, was inconsequential. The motion just was. Then I noticed another movement at the edge of what seemed to be my reassembling field of vision. This time, it was not just a component of the mechanism of physical matter but something organic, something living. A vorticella, an organism whose existence I had learned about in tenth-grade biology class.

The tulip-shaped eukaryote looks as though it ought to be multicellular but is not. I'd discovered them serendipitously in a lab experiment involving stagnant rainwater and a test tube. I felt jubilant when I viewed them under the microscope. Their long stalks, composed of protein filaments, create a recoiling molecular spring, which is triggered by exposure to calcium, yanking the flower end of the creature down toward its anchor point.

Then I felt myself breathing. I was becoming embodied. There was life after all. The sofa beneath me. The smell of cooking from an adjoining flat. Tentatively, I opened my eyes. Dazzling, vibrating light overwhelmed me. The molecules of the universe, which comprised myself, my guide, and the room, had not yet entirely reassembled. The guide came over. I squinted. I moved my lips—I had lips now—and asked, "Am I here?"

The guide sat down on the floor beside me. "Yes," they said. "You're here."

"Are you here?" I asked.

"Yes," they replied. Then, they said, "I think you're not ready to come back yet. I think you should lie down and close your eyes some more."

I reached out my hand and the guide clasped it. I lay back down, listening to the inescapable, ceaseless screeching, vibrating dissonance of the music.

Gradually, the world returned. Sounds from outside the building, regular Paris evening street noise. Cars, people's voices. A siren.

It took several minutes before I could sit up and drink some water. When I tried to describe the music to my guide, they misunderstood me at first and thought I was talking about the soundtrack they'd brought. They'd never had an auditory experience on 5-MeO-DMT. The music persisted, though intermittently and fortunately less stridently. I wanted to know how long my journey had lasted. From the time I inhaled the vapor until the time I sat up and began to speak, thirty minutes had elapsed.

We spoke for a while, then my guide had to go home. I'd arranged to speak with Mona and another friend after they left, so I did not have to process the experience alone.

I did not sleep much that night. The music persisted, intermittently, and my dreams were distorted.

The following day, ideally, would have been one in which I took long walks in a park and spoke with friends and colleagues about my experience and the nature of the universe. Instead, because I was only in Paris for a few more days, I had to spend the morning rushing about to medical imaging offices I'd recently visited to chase down documents. An administrative error on the part of the local medical authority meant I was being billed for all my scans at a ridiculous rate nonreimbursable by *la Sécu*. They'd neglected to register my move from Alsace back to Paris the year before. Where normally this kind of annoyance would cause me endless frustration bordering on anger, I found myself making my way to the practices, one of them located in a Paris neighborhood where I do not like to be, in a state of complete calm. For the first time in my life, I was entirely without anxiety. About anything. I called my guide. We talked about whether it would last.

"Neuroplasticity," they said. "It can be cultivated. It would be best if you had another session with 5-MeO in a few months."

I told them it would take me a while to get used to the idea. They suggested I take some 5-MeO-DMT back with me to the United States. In France, because it's not a scheduled drug, I couldn't be arrested for carrying it. I protested. There's the other end: the United States.

"No worries," they said. "It's synthetic. The law enforcement dogs can't detect it."

I demurred. Best to wait until I returned.

Other insights coalesced over the course of several days and weeks.

I gradually came to apprehend what I had been shown. I wanted to know the nature of life and I was shown it. In a blaze of light and sound—very much like a near-death experience, I've been told—the universe decomposed itself and then thrust me into the void so I could take the whole thing on board. Here was the universe, here were the mechanisms of the universe, here was life in the universe. And, whether I liked it or not, or whether the message was pleasant or not, I am part of it and it is part of me. There it was: the nature of being and matter staring me squarely in the face.

Contemplating this truth called to mind my experience many decades before, the night I looked into the mirror to see my naked pregnant body as it really was for the first time. That was my body. I belonged to it, it belonged to me, and other than taking my own life, there was no way to escape it. I was part of an irrefutable biological process that was, like it or not, taking place in me, and despite how much I'd been taught to hate, revile, and renounce my physical self, I could not separate from it. I was facing an unwavering, inescapable truth. I did not get to choose whether I lived in my body.

And so it is and was with me and the universe. I was presented a truth no amount of dissociation or rationalization will allow me to escape. I am of it and it is of me; we are one and the same.

And nothing—not even death or narrative—can cause the whole to separate.

ENDNOTES

Chapter 1: The Doors of Perception

1. The Consolidated Omnibus Budget Reconciliation Act confers continuing group health insurance coverage to family members under certain circumstances, divorce being one of them.
2. Arimidex is a drug in the class of aromatase inhibitors. Aromatase inhibitors arrest the cellular process by which estrogen is created in the body and are thought to prevent estrogen-receptor-positive cancer recurrence. Almost all human cells produce a tiny amount of estrogen. Aromatase inhibitors are the post-surgery and post-chemo drugs for estrogen-receptor-positive breast cancers.
3. Diane Middlebrook, *Anne Sexton: A Biography* (Vintage, 1992).

Chapter 2: The Forest and the Path

1. Jeffrey Moussaieff Masson, *The Assault on Truth: Freud's Suppression of the Seduction Theory* (Farrar, Straus and Giroux, 1984). See chapter 1: "The Aetiology of Hysteria." Freud's personal conviction, prior to his renunciation of the seduction theory, was that people, mostly women but people in general, who described being violently abused or molested as children were in fact describing real abuse at the hands of their parents or adult relatives. They were not fantasizing.

2. Michael Cornwall, "Does the Psychiatric Diagnosis Process Qualify as a Degradation Ceremony?," Mad in America, September 7, 2013, https://www.madinamerica.com/2013/09/psychiatric-diagnosis-process-qualify-degradation-ceremony/. Used with permission.

3. Charles Grob et al., "Birthing the Transpersonal," *Journal of Transpersonal Psychology* 40, no. 2 (2008): 156. Used by permission of the author.

4. *The Matrix*, written and directed by Lana Wachowski and Lilly Wachowski (Warner Brothers, 1999).

Chapter 3: Breaking Bad at Harvard

1. Munchausen syndrome by proxy is characterized by a parent or caretaker inflicting injury on a child or other dependent in order to gain attention, praise, and sympathy of medical care providers. It is a shared psychosis, a *folie à deux*, where the psychosis involves at least two people, whether they are witting or unwitting participants. My childhood psychiatrist could be described as an unwitting participant in my parents' *folie à deux*.

2. Forrest G. Robinson, *Love's Story Told: A Life of Henry A. Murray* (Harvard University Press, 1992).

3. Robinson, *Love's Story Told*.

4. Robinson, *Love's Story Told*.

5. Robinson, *Love's Story Told*.

6. Robinson, *Love's Story Told*.

7. Robinson, *Love's Story Told*.

8. Henry A. Murray, "Studies of Stressful Interpersonal Disputations," *American Psychologist* 18, no. 1 (1963): 28–36.

9. 00519Murray-Multiform-GroupIII_Dicker, archived in "Multiform Assessments of Personality Development Among Gifted College Men, 1941–1965," https://doi.org/10.7910/DVN/NKTIZD, Murray Research Archive Dataverse, V8, Harvard University.

10. Murray, "Stressful Interpersonal Disputations," 28–36.

11. Murray, "Stressful Interpersonal Disputations," 28–36.

12. Alston Chase, "A Lesson in Hate," *The Guardian*, June 21, 2000.

13. Chase, "A Lesson in Hate."

14. Robinson, *Love's Story Told*.

15. Alston Chase, "Harvard and the Making of the Unabomber," *Atlantic Monthly*, June 2000.

16. 00519Murray-Multiform_StudyDescription, archived in "Multiform Assessments of Personality Development Among Gifted College Men, 1941–1965," https://doi.org/10.7910/DVN/NKTIZD, Murray Research Archive Dataverse, V8, Murray Research Archive Dataverse, Harvard University.

17. Richard G. Adams, letter regarding Alston Chase's "Harvard and the Making of the Unabomber," Letters, *Atlantic Monthly*, September 2000.

18. Chase, "Making of the Unabomber."

19. Adams, regarding Chase's "Making of the Unabomber," 6–9.

20. Jean Delay et al., "Étude psycho-physiologique et clinique de la psilocybine," in *Les champignons hallucinogènes du Mexique*, ed. R. Heim and R. G. Wasson, (Éditions du Muséum national d'Histoire naturelle, 1958), 287–309.

21. Delay et al., "Étude psycho-physiologique," 287–309.

22. Anne-Marie Quétin, "*La psilocybine en psychiatrie clinique et expérimentale*" (thesis for the Doctorate in Medicine State Certification, Paris Faculty of Medicine, 1960).

23. See chapter 8 for a more detailed description of the roles played by Heim and Wasson and their association with the Cold War CIA operation MKULTRA.

24. Vincent Verroust, historian, oral history, from archives at the Muséum National d'Histoire Naturelle.

25. Zoë Dubus et al., "History of the Administration of Psychedelics in France," *Frontiers in Psychology* 14, no. 1 (2023).

26. Timothy Leary et al., "Americans and Mushrooms in a Naturalistic Environment: A Preliminary Report" (facsimile typescript), Houghton Library (Harvard University, 1962).

27. Rick Doblin, "Dr. Leary's Concord Prison Experiment: A 34-Year Follow-Up Study," *Journal of Psychoactive Drugs* 30, no. 4 (2008): 419–426.

28. Walter N. Pahnke, "Drugs and Mysticism: An Analysis of the Relationship Between Psychedelic Drugs and the Mystical Consciousness" (unpublished doctoral dissertation, Harvard University, 1963).

29. Pahnke, "Drugs and Mysticism," 94.

30. Pahnke, "Drugs and Mysticism," 95.

31. Pahnke, "Drugs and Mysticism," 131.

32. Thomas B. Roberts and Robert N. Jesse, "Recollections of the Good Friday Experiment: an Interview with Huston Smith," *Journal of Transpersonal Psychology* 29, no. 2 (1997).

33. R. Doblin, "Pahnke's 'Good Friday Experiment': A Long-Term Follow-Up and Methodological Critique," *Journal of Transpersonal Psychology 23, no. 1* (1991): 1–28.

34. Joseph M. Russin and Andrew T. Weil, "The Crimson Takes Leary, Alpert to Task: 'Roles' and 'Games' in William James," *Harvard Crimson,* January 24, 1963, https://www.thecrimson.com/article/1973/1/24/the-crimson-takes-leary-alpert-to/?page=1.

35. Russin and Weil, "The Crimson Takes Leary."

36. Walter N. Pahnke, "The Psychedelic Mystical Experience in the Human Encounter with Death." *Harvard Theological Review* 63, no. 1 (1969): 1–21, accessed 2021, © Cambridge University Press. Used with permission.

Chapter 4: Neurotransmitters and the Fallacy of the Magic Pill

1. Lotte C. Houtepen et al., "Genome-Wide DNA Methylation Levels and Altered Cortisol Stress Reactivity Following Childhood Trauma in Humans," *Nature Communications, March 21, 2016.*

2. Ranjani Lakshminarasimhan and Gangning Liang, "The Role of DNA Methylation in Cancer," *Advanced Experimental Medical Biology*, no. 145 (2016): 151–172.

3. James Davies, *Sedated: How Modern Capitalism Created Our Mental Health Crisis* (Atlantic Books, 2021).

4. American Psychoanalytic Association, "Getting to the Root of the Problem," posted March 12, 2018, YouTube, https://www.youtube.com/watch?v=NQCfUacxaeI, accessed August 25, 2018.

5. American Psychiatric Association, "DSM History: Post–World War II," https://www.psychiatry.org/psychiatrists/practice/dsm/about-dsm/history-of-the-dsm, accessed December 21, 2024.

6. American Psychiatric Association, "DSM History."

7. See Jeffrey Masson, *The Assault on Truth: Freud's Suppression of the Seduction Theory* (Farrar, Straus and Giroux, 1984), 55–106. In 1895, German otolaryngologist Wilhelm Fliess performed a surgery on the nasal passages of one of Freud's first analytic patients, Emma Eckstein, in order to relieve her of menstrual problems, which both men believed were caused by masturbation. Fliess, in accordance with a deranged belief that the nose and the sexual organs were intimately connected, convinced Freud that Emma's "problems" could be cured by nasal surgery. The result was catastrophic: Emma's surgical wound became infected, she became septic, and then she began hemorrhaging blood. Eventually, Freud called in another surgeon, who removed a half meter of gauze from Emma's nose left behind by Fliess during the procedure. Another hemorrhage almost killed her, and she had to be hospitalized. Although at first Freud would not absolve his colleague for the surgical malpractice, stating "we had done her an injustice; she was not at all abnormal," he later retracted the insight and declared that Emma's postoperative hemorrhages had been hysterical in nature and the result of sexual longing, all in favor of not falling out of grace with his friend.

8. American Psychiatric Association, "DSM History."

9. Peter Aldhous, "Many Authors of Psychiatry Bible Have Industry Ties," *New Scientist*, March 13, 2012.

10. Aldhous, "Many Authors."

11. *The Minority Report*, directed by Steven Spielberg (DreamWorks Pictures, 2002).

12. Davies, *Sedated*.

13. Davies, *Sedated*, 40.

14. Davies, *Sedated*, 3.

15. LSD was originally derived from one of the ergot alkaloids found in *Claviceps purpurea* and first synthesized by Albert Hoffman in 1943.

16. A. R. Green, "Gaddum and LSD: The Birth and Growth of Experimental and Clinical Neuropharmacology Research on 5-HT in the UK," *British Journal of Pharmacology* 154, no. 8 (2008): 1583–1599.

17. Bernard B. Brodie and Parkhurst A. Shore, "A Concept for a Role of Serotonin and Norepinephrine as Chemical Mediators in the Brain," *Pharmacology of Psychotomimetic and Psychotherapeutic Drugs* 66, no. 3 (1957): 631–642.

18. David Murray Shaw et al., "5-Hydroxytryptamine in the Hind-Brain of Depressive Suicides," *British Journal of Psychiatry* 113, no. 505 (1967): 1407–1411.

19. The biochemical pathway for serotonin synthesis initially involves the conversion of L-tryptophan to 5-hydroxytryptophan or 5-HT by the enzyme L-tryptophan hydroxylase (TPH). This enzyme provides the rate-limiting step for serotonin synthesis. 5-HT metabolism involves oxidation by monoamine oxidase to the corresponding aldehyde. The rate-limiting step is hydride transfer from serotonin to the flavin cofactor, which further catalyzes the aldehyde. Serotonin is metabolized in the liver to 5-HIAA, an acid waste product. At any point in either synthesis or catabolism these enzymatic functions can be disrupted by several metabolic and enzymatic factors, causing serotonin levels in the brain to fall.

20. Robert Whitaker, *Anatomy of an Epidemic: Magic Bullets, Psychiatric Drugs, and the Astonishing Rise of Mental Illness in America* (Crown Publishing, 2010).

21. Whitaker, *Anatomy*, 286.

22. Whitaker, *Anatomy*, 287.

23. Whitaker, *Anatomy*, 287.

24. Whitaker, *Anatomy*, 294.

25. Irving Kirsch, "The Emperor's New Drugs: An Analysis of Antidepressant Medication Data Submitted to the US Food and Drug Administration," *Prevention and Treatment* 5, article 23 (2002).

26. Kirsch, "The Emperor's New Drugs."

27. Kirsch, "The Emperor's New Drugs."

28. Whitaker, *Anatomy*, 335.

29. Whitaker, *Anatomy*, 335.

30. Whitaker, *Anatomy*, 335.

31. Michael P. Hengartner et al., "Antidepressant Use Prospectively Relates to a Poorer Long-Term Outcome of Depression: Results from a Prospective Community Cohort Study over 30 Years," *Psychotherapy and Psychosomatics* 87 (2018): 181–183.

32. Adele Framer, "What I Have Learnt from Helping Thousands of People Taper Off Antidepressants and Other Psychotropic Medications," *Therapeutic Advances in Psychopharmacology* 11 (2021): 1–18.

33. Rose Yesha, "Insane Medicine: How the Mental Health Industry Creates Damaging Treatment Traps and How You Can Escape Them," Mad in America, October 12, 2020, https://www.madinamerica.com. Used with permission.

34. Andrew Scull, "Thomas Insel and the Future of the Mental Health System," Mad in America, April 25, 2022, https://www.madinamerica.com/2022/04/thomas-insel-future-mental-health/. Used with permission.

35. R. Rosenheck, "The Growth of Psychopharmacology in the 1990s," *International Journal of Law and Psychiatry* 28 (2005): 467–83; US Social Security Administration, *Annual Statistical Report on the Social Security Disability Insurance Program*, 2010–2013, and *SSI Annual Statistical Report*, 2010–2013.

36. Thomas Insel, *Healing: Our Path from Mental Illness to Mental Health* (Random House, 2022).

37. Adam Rogers, "Star Neuroscientist Tom Insel Leaves the Google-Spawned Verily for . . . a Startup?" *Wired*, May 11, 2017.

38. *Letters from Generation RX,* written and directed by Kevin Miller (Journeyman Pictures, 2017).

39. Robert Whitaker, "Thomas Insel Makes a Case for Abolishing Psychiatry," Mad in America, April 30, 2022, https://www.madinamerica.com/2022/04/insel-case-abolishing-psychiatry/. Used with permission.

40. In 1963, Spanish neuroscientist José Manuel Rodriguez Delgado demonstrated how a remote-controlled brain implant could halt a charging bull in its tracks. Such a device, said Delgado, could suppress deviant behavior and be used as a means to create a "psychocivilized society." Both Elon Musk and Peter Thiel have invested heavily in intracranial implant technology.

Chapter 6: The Fate of Psycholytic Therapy in Europe

1. Alexander T. Shulgin and David E. Nichols, "Characterization of Three New Psychotomimetics," in *The Psychopharmacology of Hallucinogens*, ed. Richard C. Stillman and Robert E. Willette (Pergamon, 1978), 74–83.

2. Friederike Meckel Fischer and Ben Sessa, "Underground MDMA-, LSD- and 2-CB-Assisted Individual and Group Psychotherapy in Zurich: Outcomes, Implications and Commentary," *Drug Science, Policy and Law* 2, no. 0 (2015): 1–8, https://doi.org/10.1177/2050324515578080.

3. Fischer and Sessa, "Underground MDMA-."

4. Gerhard Roth, *Wie das Gehirn die Seele macht* (Klett-Cotta, 2014).

5. Dawn Holman et al., "The Association Between Adverse Childhood Experiences and Risk of Cancer in Adulthood: A Systematic Review of the Literature," *Pediatrics* 138, suppl. 1 (2016): 81–91, https://doi.org/10.1542/peds.2015-4268L.

Chapter 7: The Meaning of the Transpersonal

1. Charles Grob et al., "Pilot Study of Psilocybin Treatment for Anxiety in Patients with Advanced-Stage Cancer," *Archives of General Psychiatry* 68, no. 1 (2011): 71–78.
2. Erica Rex, "Calming a Turbulent Mind," *Scientific American Mind* 24, no. 2 (2013): 58–66.
3. M. Srinivasan, "Clairvoyant Remote Viewing: The US Sponsored Psychic Spying," *Strategic Analysis: A Monthly Journal of the IDSA* 26, no. 1 (2002).
4. Francesco B. DiLeo v. Catherine D. Nugent, 592 A.2d 1126 (Md. Ct. Sp. App. July 29, 1991), https://law.justia.com/cases/maryland/court-of-special-appeals/1991/644-september-term-1990-0.html.
5. Charles Grob et al., "Second Thoughts on 3,4-Methylenedioxy-methamphetamine (MDMA) Neurotoxicity," *Archives of General Psychiatry* 47, no. 3 (1990).
6. See chapter 9 for a detailed description of Dr. Grob's research with the Centro Espírita Beneficente União do Vegetal, in Brazil.

Chapter 8: The Dark Side of Psychedelics

1. Jean Delay and Philippe Benda, "L'éxperience lysergique: L.S.D.-25; À propos de 75 observations cliniques," *Encéphale* 47, no. 3 (1958).
2. Delay and Benda, "L'éxperience lysergique."
3. Delay and Benda, "L'éxperience lysergique."
4. Delay and Benda, "L'éxperience lysergique."
5. *No. de pourvoi: 94-19.685*, Cour de cassation, Chambre civile 1, du 25 février 1997, published in *Bulletin 1997* I, no. 75 (1997): 49.
6. Delay and Benda, "L'éxperience lysergique."
7. Photographed by an unidentified researcher at the French Ministry of Defense (Ministère des Armées) archive.

8. The School of the Americas was a US Army training facility established in 1946. It operated for fifty-four years, first in the Panama Canal Zone, then moving to Fort Benning in Georgia in 1984. Known by critics as the "School of the Assassins," it graduated students who went on to become some of the worst indigenous and human rights violators in the Western Hemisphere.

9. A memorandum from declassified CIA files, dated March 26, 1956, with the subject line "MKULTRA Subproject 58, Invoice #1 Allotment 6-2502-10-001," describes the underwriting of the project to collect "a hallucinogenic species of mushrooms of interest to TSS/CD." The individual whose financing was provided by Subproject 58 was "approached under the cover of the [redacted] and has applied to that organization for a grant-in-aid. He appears to be a person capable of considerable responsibility as indicated by his handling of three previous expeditions of this type and his position as vice president of [redacted]." Wasson was, at the time, *vice president* for public relations at J.P. Morgan & Company. Further pages consist of Wasson's grant application, which describes a person who will accompany him on the trip: "Professor [redacted], leading mycologist and Director of the [redacted] has committed himself to accompany me on this trip. His great experience in mycology generally and in tropical mycology in particular will be of very great value." The professor was Dr. Roger Heim, director of the French Museum of Natural History and director of the laboratory for the study of mycology and tropical phytopathology at the École Pratique des Hautes Études in Paris.

10. Jean Delay et al., "Étude psycho-physiologique et clinique de la psilocybine," in *Les champignons hallucinogènes du Mexique*, ed. R. Heim and R. G. Wasson, (Éditions du Muséum National d'Histoire Naturelle, 1958), 287–309.

11. Anne-Marie Quétin, "*La psilocybine en psychiatrie clinique et expérimentale*," (thesis for the Doctorate in Medicine State Certification, Paris Faculty of Medicine, 1960).

12. Lily Kay Ross and David Nickles, hosts, *Power Trip*, podcast, produced by *New York* magazine and Psymposia, 2021–2022, https://www.psymposia.com/powertrip/. Used with permission.

13. Allison Feduccia, "Can We Quantify the Placebo Effect in Psychedelic Medicine?" Psychedelic Support, March 1, 2019, https://psyche-delic.support/resources/placebo-effect-psychedelics-medicine/.

14. Ross and Nickles, *Power Trip*.

15. Hanna Rosin, "You Won't Feel High After Watching This Video," *New York*, March 22, 2022.

16. Lily Kay Ross and David Nickles, "The Trials of Rick Doblin: He Revolutionized the Way We View MDMA-Assisted Psychotherapy. But What Does the Research Actually Show?" *New York*, May 11, 2022.

17. Ross and Nickles, "Trials of Rick Doblin."

18. Ross and Nickles, "Trials of Rick Doblin."

Chapter 9: The Culture Is the Medicine / The Culture Is the Poison

1. Deborah Bassett et al., "'Our Culture Is Medicine': Perspectives of Native Healers on Posttraumatic Recovery Among American Indian and Alaska Native Patients," *Permanente Journal* 16, no. 1 (2012).

2. Allison Feduccia, "Can We Quantify the Placebo Effect in Psychedelic Medicine?" Psychedelic Support, March 1, 2019, https://psyche-delic.support/resources/placebo-effect-psychedelics-medicine/.

3. According to verbal reports from former BPRU staff, at least two people attempted suicide. One killed himself following his first session, having declared he was quitting the study because he felt the treatment wasn't working. Roland Griffiths dismissed the data, claiming the suicide did not count as an adverse event, as the subject was no longer in the study when his death occurred.

4. John Elflein, "Total Number of Cases and Deaths from COVID-19 in the United States as of April 26, 2023," Statista,

August 29, 2023, https://www.statista.com/statistics/1101932/coronavirus-covid19-cases-and-deaths-number-us-americans/.

5.   Christian Angermayer (@C_Angermayer), "To go on with complete shut down for more than 2 wks is absurd and violating any civil rights we fought for," Twitter (now X), March 18, 2020, https://www.psymposia.com/magazine/christian-angermayer-coronavirus-capitalism. Used with permission.

6.   Plus Three, "Amidst Pandemic, Psychedelic Investor Christian Angermayer Can't Imagine Life Beyond Capitalism," Psymposia, April 4, 2020, https://www.psymposia.com/magazine/christian-angermayer-coronavirus-capitalism. Used with permission.

7.   Glen Adams et al., "The Psychology of Neoliberalism and the Neoliberalism of Psychology," *Journal of Social Issues* 75, no. 1 (2019): 189–216.

8.   Sarah Riley et al., "Turn On, Tune In, but Don't Drop Out: The Impact of Neo-Liberalism on Magic Mushroom Users' (In) Ability to Imagine Collectivist Social Worlds," *International Journal of Drug Policy* 21, no. 6 (2010): 445–451.

9.   Charles Grob and Marlene Dobkin de Rios, "Adolescent Drug Use in Cross-Cultural Perspective," *Journal of Drug Issues* 22, no. 1 (1992): 121–138. Used with permission.

10. Grob and Dobkin de Rios, "Adolescent Drug Use."

11. Grob and Dobkin de Rios, "Adolescent Drug Use."

12. Grob and Dobkin de Rios, "Adolescent Drug Use."

13. Marlene Dobkin de Rios, *The Psychedelic Journey of Marlene Dobkin de Rios: 45 Years with Shamans, Ayahuasqueros, and Ethnobotanists* (Park Street Press, 2009).

14. Dobkin de Rios, *The Psychedelic Journey.*

15. Charles Grob et al., "Human Psychopharmacology of Hoasca, a Plant Hallucinogen Used in Ritual Context in Brazil," *Journal of Nervous and Mental Disease* 184, no. 2 (1996): 86–94. Used with permission of the authors.

16. Grob et al., "Human Psychopharmacology of Hoasca."

17. Grob et al., "Human Psychopharmacology of Hoasca."

18. Erowid, "Legal Status of Ayahuasca in Brazil," The Vaults of Erowid, March 2001, https://erowid.org/chemicals/ayahuasca/ ayahuasca_law6.shtml.

19. Grob et al., "Human Psychopharmacology of Hoasca."

20. Grob et al., "Human Psychopharmacology of Hoasca."

21. Grob et al., "Human Psychopharmacology of Hoasca."

22. Jeremy Narby, "Living Responsibly in the Biosphere," transcript of keynote at *National Bioneers Conference, 2017, posted February 13, 2018,* https://bioneers.org/jeremy-narby-living-responsibly -biosphere-ztvz1802/.

Epilogue: Seeing What Is There

1. *"Qui sommes-nous?"* Société Psychédélique Française, accessed Jan 17, 2024, https://societepsychedelique.fr/fr/qui-sommes-nous. The society is dedicated to the exploration and dissemination of scientific and cultural information about psychedelics, as well as providing a hub for students and researchers interested in interdisciplinary collaboration. The society provides a friendly community for users in the spirit of responsibility and risk reduction.

2. See chapter 9 for a detailed description of dimethyltryptamine, DMT. 5-methoxy-N,N-dimethyltryptamine or 5-MeO-DMT was first identified by toxicologist Dr. Vittorio Erspamer, whose most important contribution to neuroscience was the identification and synthesis of the neurotransmitter serotonin. He was interested in the exudate from amphibian parotid glands as a possible source of new medical drugs. He analyzed the venom from forty toad species. One species, *Incilius alvarius,* the Sonoran Desert toad, was found to synthesize a DMT-containing substance, 5-MeO-DMT. The discovery of 5-MeO-DMT in the glands of the Sonoran Desert toad led to widespread poaching in the southwestern United States, threatening the species' survival. The substance is safely and easily formulated in a laboratory. The

5-MeO-DMT that I vaped was laboratory formulated and had been sourced in Belgium.

3. Sarah Jefferson et al., "5-MeO-DMT Modifies Innate Behaviors and Promotes Structural Neural Plasticity in Mice," *Neuropsychopharmacology* 48 (2023): 1257–1266; Rafael Victor Lima da Cruz et al., "Corrigendum: A Single Dose of 5-MeO-DMT Stimulates Cell Proliferation, Neuronal Survivability, Morphological and Functional Changes in Adult Mice Ventral Dentate Gyrus," *Frontiers in Molecular Neuroscience* 11, article 312 (2018).

4. I've since identified the pattern as resembling the tile composition found in the mosque at Isfahan.

5. Mona Sobhani, *Proof of Spiritual Phenomena: A Neuroscientist's Discovery of the Ineffable Mysteries of the Universe* (Park Street Press, 2022).

ACKNOWLEDGMENTS

There are numerous beings, human and nonhuman, without whose efforts this book would never have been written. First among these, Nadine Rubin Nathan, book agent, champion of real writing, and tireless reader of drafts; Mike Oreskes, for encouragement, excellent editorial input, and sage counsel; Stephen Mills, whose wisdom guided my writing about trauma; Sarah Alfadl, for help and friendship over the course of many decades; and Tom Watkins, whose unflagging encouragement—and flagging of citation errors—made this a better book. Thanks also to Dr. Robin Carhart-Harris, whose doctoral research launched me on this journey; Dr. Charles Grob, Dr. Anthony Bossis, Dr. David Nutt, and Robert Whitaker, who encouraged me to complete the draft. Thank you also to Andy Reinhardt, whose Paris home provided a safe harbor during the COVID-19 pandemic lockdown, where much of this book was written.

I would also like to express my gratitude to those whose sensitivity, claircognizance, and intuition helped me find my way back into my own body: the instructors at Bay Area Model Mugging in the early 1990s; my riding teachers, Judy Brawley, Bob Brawley, and Steve Newell; and the horses who were my teachers: Scarlet Wakeena, Brown County, Sportin' Life, Kind of Blue, and Clapton. And lastly, perhaps most importantly, Keo, Swedish Vallhund extraordinaire, 2005–2023, dog on a mission, mind reader, protector. Thank you.

ABOUT THE AUTHOR

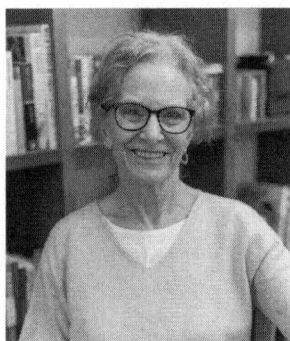

E rica Rex's journalism and essays have been published in *The New York Times*, *The Times* (*Eureka Science Magazine*), *The Independent*, *Scientific American*, *Scientific American Mind*, *Poets & Writers*, and others. Her fiction has appeared in *The North American Review*, *Promethean*, and others. She speaks frequently about psychedelics, society, and medicine on the *Psychedelics Today* podcast. She is an advisor to the United States Congressional Caucus Protecting Public Health and Safety with Psychedelics Advancing Therapies (PATH). She is an American Society of Magazine Editors award-winning fiction writer and a fellow of the MacDowell Colony, the Ucross Foundation, and the Helene Wurlitzer Foundation. Her constant companion, a Swedish Vallhund named Luna, keeps her on her toes, reminding her that the beach is an indispensable component of a life well lived and that the use of electronic devices before sleep is a recipe for anxiety. Erica (and Luna) divide their time between the United Kingdom, Europe, and the United States.

Author photo © Jason Gardner

Looking for your next great read?

We can help!

Visit www.shewritespress.com/next-read
or scan the QR code below for a list
of our recommended titles.

She Writes Press is an award-winning
independent publishing company founded to
serve women writers everywhere.

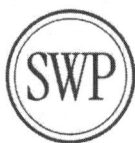